MAKE MOVEMENT
YOUR
MEDICINE

For our children Theo and Orianne Breakspear for
encouraging and supporting us always.

To all our patients and Pilates groups
with whom we have worked to create the
Breakspear Make Movement Your Medicine method.

MAKE MOVEMENT YOUR MEDICINE

Gentle Exercises to Soothe and Revive Your Upper Back, Neck and Shoulders

ANDY & RACHEL BREAKSPEAR

BLOOMSBURY SPORT
LONDON · OXFORD · NEW YORK · NEW DELHI · SYDNEY

BLOOMSBURY SPORT
Bloomsbury Publishing Plc
50 Bedford Square, London, WC1B 3DP, UK
Bloomsbury Publishing Ireland Limited,
29 Earlsfort Terrace, Dublin 2, D02 AY28, Ireland

BLOOMSBURY, BLOOMSBURY SPORT and the Diana logo are trademarks of Bloomsbury Publishing Plc

First published in Great Britain 2026

Copyright © Andy Breakspear and Rachel Breakspear, 2026
Photography © Henry Hunt with the exception of the following: pp. 8, 9, 18, 21, 22, 24, 25, 30, 31 and 32
© Getty Images

Andy Breakspear and Rachel Breakspear have asserted their right under the Copyright, Designs and Patents Act, 1988, to be identified as Authors of this work

For legal purposes the Acknowledgements on p. 176 constitute an extension of this copyright page

All rights reserved. No part of this publication may be: i) reproduced or transmitted in any form, electronic or mechanical, including photocopying, recording or by means of any information storage or retrieval system without prior permission in writing from the publishers; or ii) used or reproduced in any way for the training, development or operation of artificial intelligence (AI) technologies, including generative AI technologies. The rights holders expressly reserve this publication from the text and data mining exception as per Article 4(3) of the Digital Single Market Directive (EU) 2019/790

Bloomsbury Publishing Plc does not have any control over, or responsibility for, any third-party websites referred to or in this book. All internet addresses given in this book were correct at the time of going to press. The author and publisher regret any inconvenience caused if addresses have changed or sites have ceased to exist, but can accept no responsibility for any such changes. The material contained in this book is for informational purposes only. No material in this publication is intended to be a substitute for professional medical advice, diagnosis or treatment. Always seek the advice of your GP or other qualified health care professional with any questions you may have regarding a medical condition, including mental health concerns, or treatment and before undertaking a new healthcare regime, and never disregard professional medical advice or delay in seeking it because of something you have read in this book.

Please note: While every effort has been made to ensure that the contents of this book are as safe and effective as possible, neither the authors nor the publishers can accept responsibility for any injury or loss sustained as a result of the use of this material.

A catalogue record for this book is available from the British Library

Library of Congress Cataloguing-in-Publication data has been applied for

ISBN: PB: 978-1-3994-1862-1; ePUB: 978-1-3994-1861-4; ePDF: 978-1-3994-1859-1

Typeset in Sofia Pro by D.R. Ink
Printed and bound in China by C&C Offset Printing Co., Ltd.

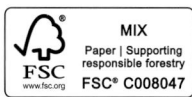

To find out more about our authors and books visit www.bloomsbury.com and sign up for our newsletters
For product safety related questions contact productsafety@bloomsbury.com

CONTENTS

Foreword	6
How to use this book	7
PART 1 BACK TO BASICS	**12**
1. Introducing the Make Movement Your Medicine method	14
2. Why modern living is a strain	20
3. Understanding how your body moves	28
4. How to achieve good posture	34
5. Tightness tests	41
PART 2 EXERCISES AND SEQUENCES	**54**
6. Upper back movements, stretches and self-massages	56
7. Neck movements, stretches and self-massages	78
8. Shoulder movements, stretches and self-massages	93
9. Targeted exercise combinations	114
Glossary	172
About us	173
The Adjuvo™ massage and mobility pole	173
Directory of movements, stretches and self-massages	174
Directory of exercise combinations	175
Acknowledgements	176

FOREWORD

Upper back, neck and shoulder pain are among the most common consequences of modern life. Too often the medical solutions offered are passive: medication, rest, or simply learning to endure. What Andy and Rachel offer here is active empowerment by daily preventive exercises, short and frequent, to do at work and home.

This book is built on a simple truth: movement heals. With clear explanations and step-by-step guidance, the Breakspears show how anyone can restore mobility, reduce pain and prevent recurring problems. What makes their approach so valuable is its accessibility – you don't need special equipment or advanced fitness, only the willingness to explore what movement can do. We all know how hard discipline is! Daily implementation of these sitting and standing exercises will keep you vital for longer and this is exactly what we recommend to our patients and staff.

    As occupational physicians, we know that knowledge becomes medicine when it is applied. This book turns knowledge into action, and action into lasting health. We wholeheartedly commend this book to you and urge everyone to read it.

Dr Herman Spanjaard, MD, MPH, FACOEM, International Occupational Health Consultant, and **Dr Richard JL Heron**, MB ChB FRCP FFOM FFOMI FACOEM, Independent Chief Medical Officer

HOW TO USE THIS BOOK

In a world where many people spend their days sitting down in front of a computer, hunched over a phone or being otherwise sedentary, the number of people who suffer with upper back, neck and shoulder pain has increased, and the age at which people first experience problems has dropped. What was once an ailment common mostly among the older population has become an issue that now also affects children, teenagers and younger adults.

So, aside from moving more and spending less time on screens, what can people do to alleviate these all-too-common aches and pains? Fortunately, the answer is, quite a lot.

Make Movement Your Medicine is a comprehensive collection of exercises and self-massages that, in this book, focus on the upper back, neck and shoulders. The aim of this book is to help those areas of your body function comfortably and freely, and to regain and retain their full range of motion. The good news is that doing this requires neither a lot of time nor money. You don't need to go to a gym or own lots of fancy equipment: we have ensured that the movements in this book can be done sitting down or standing up, at any time, in any location, and with no (or only minimal) special equipment (*see* p. 10 for more on equipment).

Because each exercise takes only a minute or two, you can do them regularly, whenever it's convenient. You could practise a few every time you make a cup of tea or coffee, before you put your shoes on or each time you have a meal. You can set an hourly alarm to remind you to take a one- or two-minute movement break or you could block off five minutes between meetings to do a few exercises.

Over time, making movement your medicine will become an automatic habit, as natural as washing your hands or sipping a drink. Even better if you can persuade others to join in with you, too. Research shows that if you get someone to exercise with you, your consistency improves, and of course, it means they also reap the benefits. The same is true if you choose a set time every day to exercise, for example before you have breakfast or each time you have a drink, even if it is only for a minute.

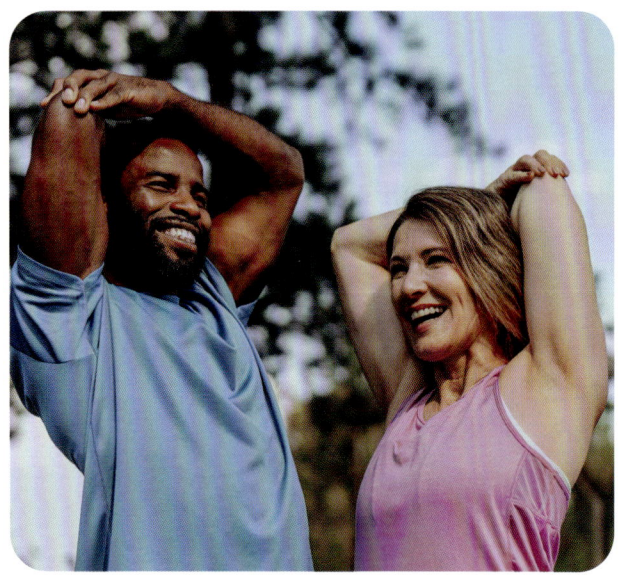

RELIEF ROADMAP

To enhance the ease and speed of making movement a habit and relieving everyday niggles, this book has been designed so that you can dip into it and quickly find the appropriate movement, stretch or massage. We suggest you have a look through the chapters in Part 1 when you first read the book, because they set the context for the movements, describe our method, advise on good posture, and explain how to test how tight your body is, but you don't need to read them every time. In the future, you could jump straight to the tightness tests in Chapter 5 (*see* pp. 42–53). These are arranged by area – upper back, neck and shoulders – and will allow you to assess where the problem lies. Depending on your results, you will be able to head straight to the exercises that tackle the identified issue.

These exercises are all contained in Part 2 of the book, with separate chapters for the upper back (*see* pp. 56–77), neck (*see* pp. 78–92) and shoulders (*see* pp. 93–113) to help you hone in on the problem area. You don't have to do all of the exercises at once or in any particular order, though it's worth doing the Essential warm-up exercises before you begin (*see* Table 9.1 on p. 116). Experiment and see which ones you find most effective and enjoyable and perhaps bookmark them. If you know you are prone to having a stiff upper back after sitting at a desk all day, or often wake up with a sore neck, then you can flick to the relevant exercises and access relief strategies. This targeted approach not only helps you identify and tackle the problem quickly, but it should stop you feeling overwhelmed and may make it easier to incorporate movement into your daily routine.

You may also wish to customise and combine your chosen therapeutic movements, stretches and self-massages, depending on the time you have available, the area of your body you want to focus on and what you like doing. We guide you to easily do this in Chapter 9 (*see* pp. 114–171, which contains ready-made exercise combinations. These remove the guesswork and ensure you are making best use of your time. For example, if you are an office worker with a stiff upper back, turn to table 9.8 on p. 130 for a sequence of simple exercises you can do at your desk. If you're gardening and want to stave off the aches and stiffness that are common after that activity, turn to table 9.15 on p. 144. All sorts of different scenarios are covered, from sequences for new parents, manual labourers and travellers through to sport-specific action plans (*see* p. 175 for a complete list of exercise combinations).

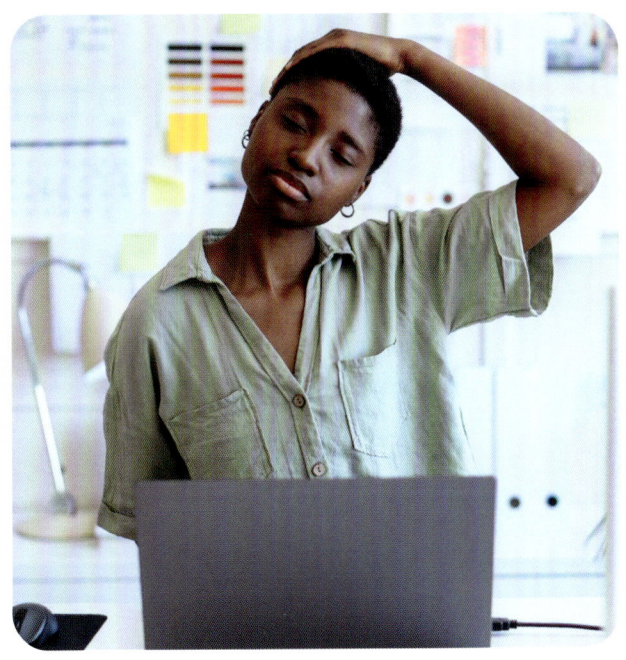

AT-A-GLANCE GUIDE

- Flick to p. 35 for notes on good posture.
- Flick to pp. 30–3 to understand how the upper back, shoulders and neck work.
- Flick to Chapter 5 to find the tightness tests and discover which movements, stretches and self-massages you could begin with to tackle a particular area of tightness.
- Flick to Chapters 6, 7 and 8 for step-by-step instructions on how to do the movements, stretches and self-massages.
- Flick to Chapter 9 for ready-made combinations and sequences of movements, stretches and self-massages.

Of course, if you prefer to explore the content in detail first you can also read the book from cover to cover, and if you'd rather work through it doing all the movements, stretches and self-massages in the chapters in Part 2, then that's perfectly fine, too. However, it is the practice of regular movement that is most important. You can make progress by working on the exercises for 15 to 20 minutes three times a week, but you can also get great benefits by moving, stretching and self-massaging for just a few minutes several times a day, perhaps once an hour. That's what we recommend, but equally we always say that some movement is better than none, so just do what you can manage.

Correcting poor posture is a habit we also wholeheartedly recommend, and we have provided a whole chapter on this foundational aspect of good upper back, neck and shoulder health on pp. 34–40. Are you prone to slumping as you sit at a desk? If that's you, turn to the instructions on how to sit with neutral posture on p. 39. Do you slouch or put most of your weight through one leg? Check out the advice on how to stand tall on p. 35. There's even guidance on how to improve your breathing on p. 38 and the best way to look down on pp. 26–27. We firmly believe that teaching your body to adopt good posture is one of the best ways to minimise issues cropping up in the first place, and together with regular movement, can transform your life.

But don't just take our word for it. We have treated countless patients over the years, and some of them have been kind enough to allow us to use their words in this book to describe how our approach has helped them. These stories reveal the power of movement and how small changes can make a big difference, sometimes even removing the need for surgery.

HOW TO MOVE SAFELY

Although this book is intended to help you help yourself, it is important to stress that if you are experiencing acute or prolonged pain, it is very important to consult a medical practitioner. The same is true if you have certain pre-existing conditions, such as severe arthritis, scoliosis, herniated or bulging disc, osteoporosis, previous spinal surgery, cancer and other conditions besides.

If it is appropriate to exercise, care still needs to be taken when performing the movements, stretches and self-massages outlined in this book, and when testing for tightness. We sometimes talk about 'working towards pain'. What we mean by this is gently approaching a point of discomfort but not continuing to where you feel increasing or sharp pain. You should not work through pain. The most you should feel is moderate discomfort. Listen to your body and stop when discomfort tips over into pain. It is best to be cautious and seek professional advice if you are unsure of how to proceed or want additional support.

If you are in pain or have restricted movement but are able to exercise, you can try any exercise or self-massage in a mini or even a micro version while your body is rehabilitating. That said, you shouldn't push yourself to continue or get very tired, nor do anything that increases the pain, so if even doing a micro version of any of the movements, stretches or self-massages hurts, stop and seek medical guidance.

The aim of our work, and of this book, is to get your body moving so you can correct any issues and include more health-enhancing upper body movement in your daily routine. We believe that once you've tried some of these techniques you'll quickly notice how much better you feel and be emboldened to truly make movement your medicine, for life.

WHO WE ARE

Before we go any further, we want to explain who we are, and why we are qualified to provide this advice. We are a husband-and-wife team of professionals with medical expertise and decades of experience. Andy is a registered osteopath and Rachel is an advanced movement therapist. For the past 30 years we have run a clinic helping people to live free of muscle and joint pain. We work with patients of all ages and abilities, including doctors, international athletes and even a *Strictly Come Dancing* contestant! We are also teachers and passionate about empowering people to look after their bodies in just a few minutes each day.

A NOTE ON EQUIPMENT

For many of the movements in this book you don't need any equipment at all, but for others, a few everyday items or easily accessible equipment can be helpful.

The first of these is a long, smooth pole, such as a strong broom handle or dowel, which is used for exercises and massage. If you need additional height, you may need to place the pole on a stable stool or something similar.

A fixed item such as a doorframe, horizontal beam or a secure pull-up bar can be used for stretching and assisted hanging but be careful not to strain your hands or fingers. Alternatively, you could use monkey bars at a local park or playground.

A long towel or strong strap looped over a secure beam is another way of improvising a set-up for movement and stretching, although it won't give you the rigidity required for optimum results. Still, it's better than nothing, and does work. For the therapeutic movements you need a pole that you can move.

A slim massage roller is ideal for self-massages if you have one, but you can also use things you probably already have at home. A plastic water bottle filled with water and then frozen can become a massage roller, as can a rolling pin or pieces of PVC pipe, although you may need to cushion these with a towel. You could make a softer tube massage roller by cutting to size a solid foam tube, such as a swimming noodle. A tennis ball in a sock can also be useful for targeting small areas of the shoulders, upper back and neck.

Since we, as medical practitioners, need to use equipment every day, we designed our own massage and mobility pole with an integral massage roller, called the Adjuvo™ pole. For information on this, *see* p. 173.

THE BENEFITS OF USING A POLE

Working with a pole offers several therapeutic advantages, especially when you're exercising alone:

- **Versatile:** You can stand or sit when you're exercising, making the exercises available to everyone, from ninja warriors to those needing to exercise while seated.
- **Movement coach:** Like a coach, a pole helps to ensure alignment of your body as you move, giving you the confidence to know your form is correct and safe.
- **Unique hanging stretches:** A pole enables powerful hanging stretches to promote shoulder comfort and health, which can be performed standing or sitting.
- **Shoulder-problem friendly:** Even if your shoulders are currently painful or have restricted movement, a pole will support the weight of your arms during exercises, so your shoulders can benefit from performing a greater range of pain-free movement.
- **Exercise enhancer:** Exercising with a pole can provide extra resistance or assistance with balance and co-ordination.

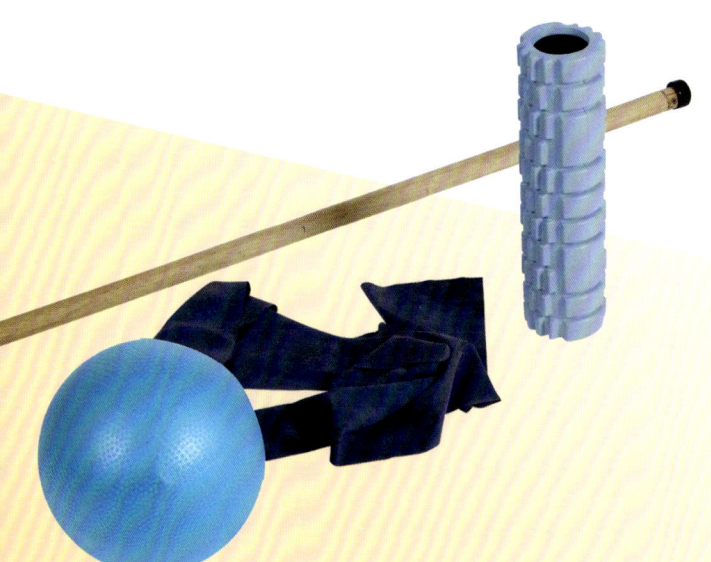

PART 1

BACK TO BASICS

The number of people experiencing upper back, neck and shoulder pain has increased significantly in recent years. Most people with these symptoms used to be middle-aged or older, but there has been a sharp rise in people in their 20s and 30s needing osteopathic treatment for upper body pain. Even more shockingly, growing numbers of parents are seeking treatment for their children, some of whom are as young as five, because they have neck pain.

So, what's going on, and what can you do to help yourself?

The answer to both questions is movement – a lack of it for the former and doing more of it for the latter.

In this section, in Chapter 1 we will first explain the ideology and core principles of our Make Movement Your Medicine method: how it works, what it involves, and who it is for. This sets out our stall, as it were, and clarifies the ethos at the heart of the book.

In Chapter 2, we take a deep dive into the root causes of the issues we see time and time again in our clinics and examine how modern life is affecting our bodies. We've included a few quick fixes here that will instantly improve your body positioning while carrying out everyday tasks, such as looking down at a screen, a phone – or even this book!

Chapter 3 examines in more detail how our bodies work and move, so that you can better understand the structure of the body parts this book talks about, and why they can go wrong.

Chapter 4 contains the key to preventing issues occurring in the first place: improving posture. Here we provide step-by-step guidance to improving how you stand, sit and breathe.

Chapter 5 is all about testing for tightness and will enable you to identify and self-diagnose areas of tension and pain in the upper back, neck and shoulders. Armed with this information, you can then select appropriate exercises from Part 2 to alleviate the problem.

1 INTRODUCING THE MAKE MOVEMENT YOUR MEDICINE METHOD

Make Movement Your Medicine is a self-help method that we have developed over 30 years of working with patients in our clinic. Providing fast relief from aches and pains in the muscles and joints of the upper body, it has enabled patients to be more physically able, feel younger and live a pain-free life. Now we want to share our knowledge and do the same for you, relieving existing problems as well as helping you avoid issues in the future.

Our approach has three components:

1. **Therapeutic movements**
2. **Stretches (including unique hanging stretches using a pole)**
3. **Self-massage**

All of these are based on sound scientific principles and research and have been tried and tested. They work in a complementary way, so each component enhances the effect of the others to give optimum relief with minimum effort.

Given how important they are, it's worth taking a moment to look at each component more closely.

1. Therapeutic movements

These movements are designed to reduce pain, and activate, loosen and improve muscle function. They help your muscles work together and prevent them from becoming stiff, weak and painful, which reduces the risk of injury or loss of movement. They also have a lubricating effect and enable you to move your joints and muscles through their full range of natural motion, so you stay maximally nimble and flexible.

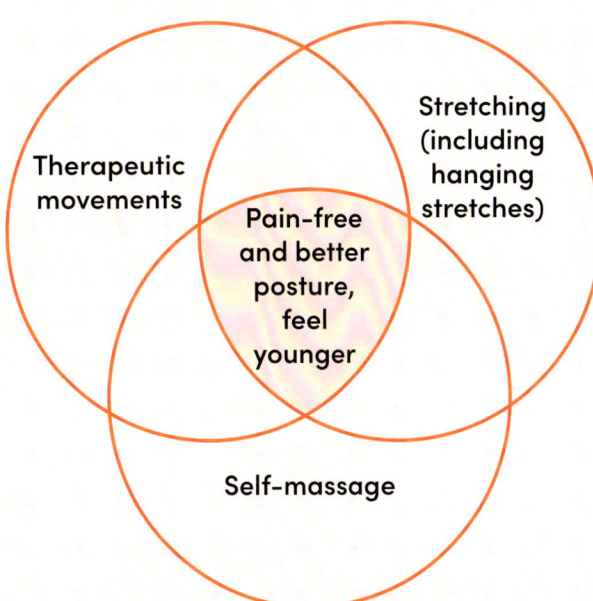

THE IMPORTANCE OF UPPER BACK MOBILITY

Over the last 30 years, more than 90 per cent of all the upper back, neck and shoulder problems we have treated in our clinic have had one common factor: upper back tightness. This places excess work and strain on the neck and shoulders.

The fact is, if you want your upper back, neck and shoulders to remain comfortable and to function properly, upper back mobility is crucial. This means that you need to release any tightness in the area on a daily basis. This might sound daunting, but the good news is that it is easily achieved by doing three simple movements – rotation, flexion/extension and side arcing. Let's take a quick look at what these are:

1. Rotation is gently twisting or turning your upper back/spine to one side and then the other.
2. Flexion/extension is forward and backward bending of your upper back/spine.
3. Side bending/arcing is curving your upper back/spine to one side and then the other.

These three simple movements, which can all be done sitting or standing, are the best way to ensure you address the main underlying cause of your aches and pains, rather than just relieving the symptoms. We firmly believe that anyone, regardless of age, can improve their physical functioning and well-being just by incorporating these three movements into their day. For this reason, you will find that all three are included in all of the targeted exercise combinations in Chapter 9.

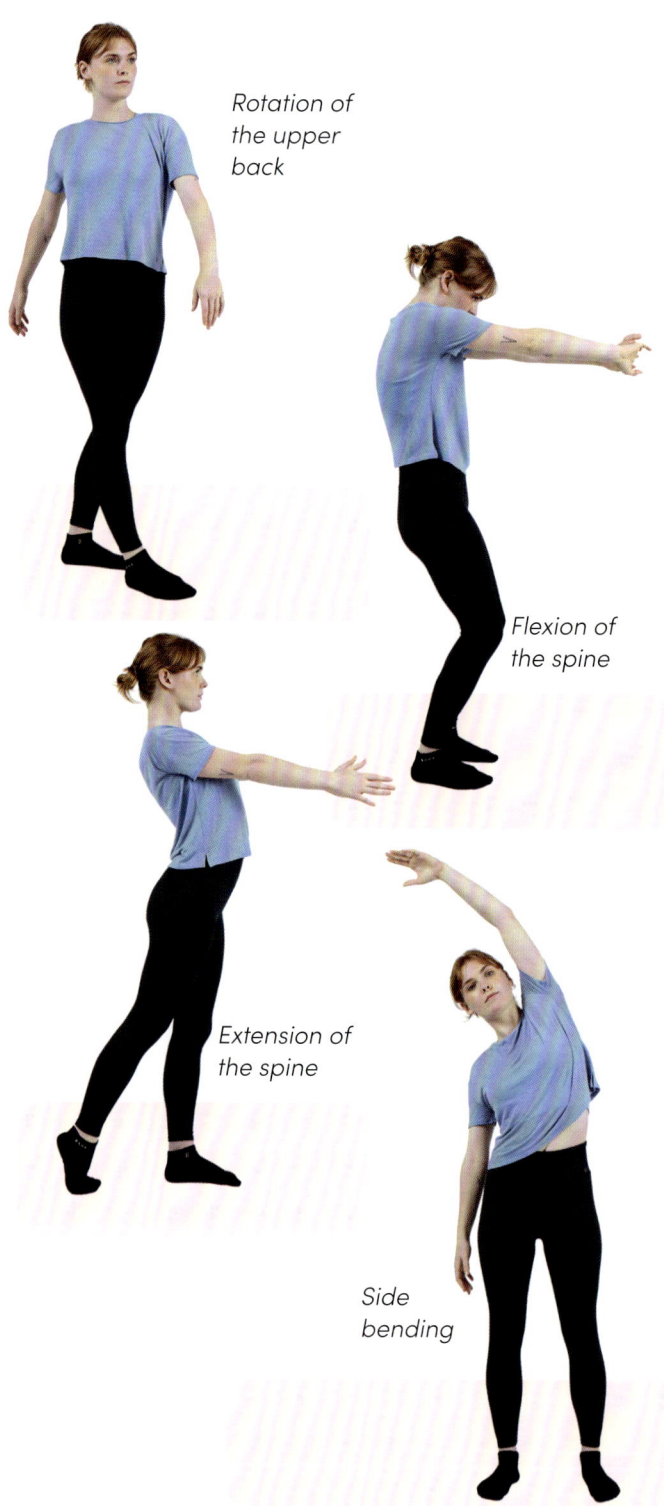

Rotation of the upper back

Flexion of the spine

Extension of the spine

Side bending

2. Stretches

Stretches are very good for your posture: they improve your flexibility, take pressure off your joints, and reduce tightness and pain. Stretching your muscles also improves blood flow and ensures your joints retain their full range of movement. This in turn improves co-ordination and body control, encouraging mental clarity and relaxation.

There are many ways of doing stretches – static (stationary), dynamic (moving), isometric (holding) and others – but we particularly favour using assisted hanging stretches from a pole for the upper back and shoulders (see pp. 104–7). These provide a really strong stretching effect in a safe and effective way and with variables that you can control. You can do these either standing or sitting, and the intensity of the hangs can be easily adjusted by changing the positioning of your hand and altering the amount of weight being placed on the pole. This ensures your upper back and shoulders can be comfortable while still gaining the benefits of hanging.

Furthermore, research shows that that like other primates, humans are meant to use their arms for climbing and hanging, and that we need these natural movements to maintain a comfortable upper body. Unless you are a climber, a gymnast or a child who enjoys the monkey bars or climbing frames, few of us do much climbing or hanging in our regular lives.

We want to change that. Our assisted hanging stretches really open up your joints and release tight muscles and soft tissues, to improve and maintain your natural range of movement. The forward, side and cross hang stretches also give wonderful release in the upper back, particularly between the shoulder blades.

HOW WE DEVELOPED ASSISTED HANGING STRETCHES

Andy hurt his shoulder in a skiing accident and it soon became apparent that he had done some significant damage – not good for an osteopath who needs fully functioning shoulders. He had surgery and faced three months of rehabilitation but was determined to find a way to maximise the results.

While walking in nearby woods, Andy noticed a hornbeam bough growing at an angle across the path. Using his strong arm he lifted his post-operative arm as high as he could without pain and held on to the branch. By slowly lowering his body Andy began partially hanging from the tree. His shoulder muscles initially felt slightly sore, because the tightness in them needed to be released. He was careful to avoid sharp pain, but his shoulder quickly started to ease, and he felt a significant improvement in its range of movement and strength.

Inspired by Andy's experience, and by experimenting and working with patients in our clinic, we developed a series of assisted hanging stretches that use a pole instead of a tree branch. This makes these exercises available to all and it also enables controlled assisted hanging to be done while standing or sitting.

Note: It is important to approach assisted hanging with a pole gently, to prevent excessive soreness.

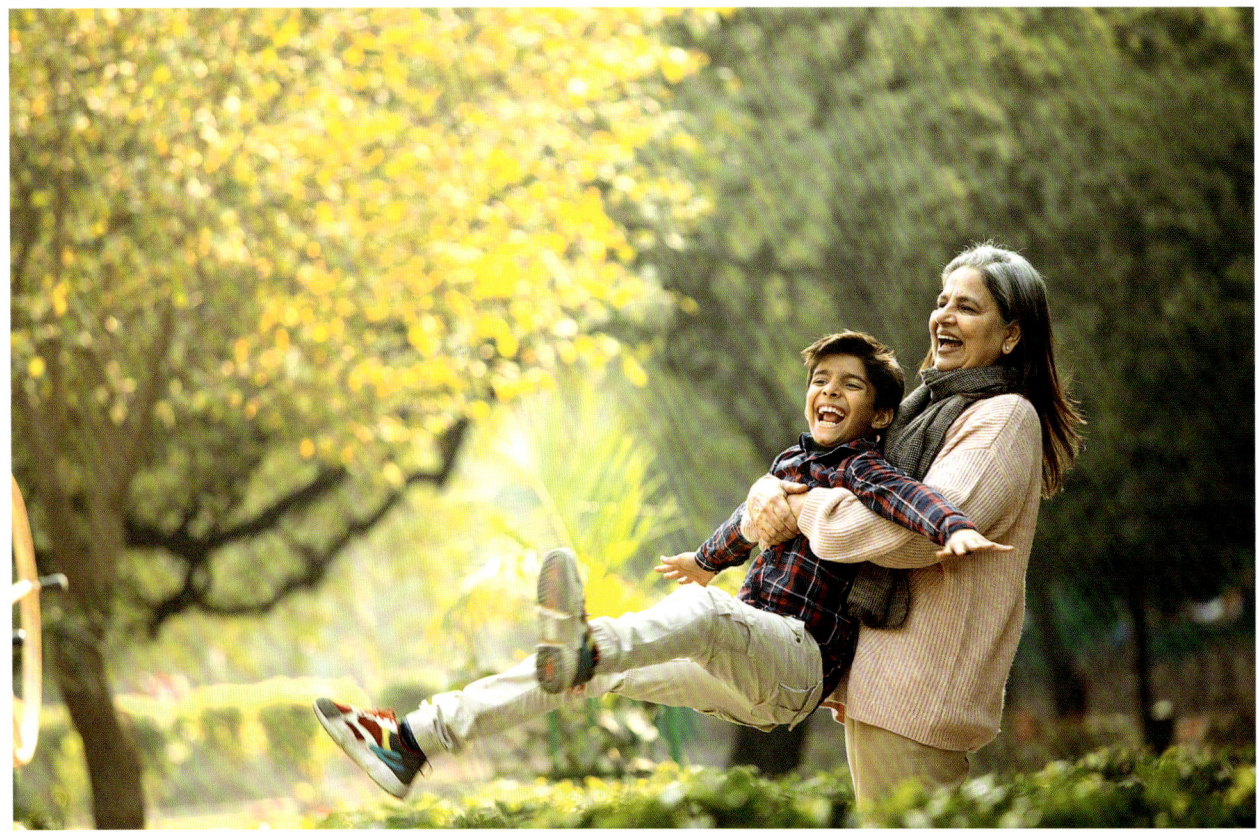

3. Self-massage

By focusing on specific points where your muscles can become tight, self-massage complements the other two components. It provides muscular pain relief, eases local muscle tension, increases circulation by improving blood flow to your muscles, and promotes relaxation and recovery by stimulating or calming the tissues and nerve endings. It can also reduce inflammation, keeping your muscles healthy and comfortable, and can alleviate headaches and tension caused by hours of screen time.

In cases of simple muscle soreness or stiffness, which can happen when areas of muscle become 'stuck', self-massage can help you to release the contraction and bring about an immediate improvement in function. You can then use the movements and stretches to maintain your mobility, returning occasionally to self-massage different areas as required, just like a bear rubbing its back on a tree.

> **EXERCISE SYMBOLS**
>
> To help you identify whether an exercise needs any equipment, we have included a **P** symbol for stretches that require a pole, and an **R** symbol for self-massages that require a roller.

WHO THIS BOOK IS FOR

Anyone who wants to know how to take care of their upper back, neck and shoulders, regardless of age or fitness level, will find this book beneficial. All the movements are useful for both preventing issues from arising and for easing any existing issues. Most only take a minute or so to do, and they're all tried, tested and safe.

This book is for you if you spend most of your day at a desk or frequently use a smartphone, laptop or tablet. Or perhaps you're living with a health condition such as arthritis or scoliosis and want a simple self-help method to manage it. You might have a sports injury or be recovering from joint surgery and be seeking exercises you can do without getting down on the floor. Or maybe you are looking to improve your range of movement so you can stay agile and avoid aches and pains.

When you are in pain, your quality of life suffers. Our Make Movement Your Medicine method can help to lower the level of pain you experience, reducing your reliance on regular pain-control medication. With time, you may even find that it allows you to not only become pain-free, but to *stay* pain-free, with no negative side-effects.

Whatever your reason for picking this book up, it will help you understand what good posture is, why it matters (*see* p. 35), and how to gain and maintain it via quick and easy exercises (*see* pp. 164–5). Straightforward, practical and designed for immediate use, these movements, stretches and self-massage routines will help you manage tension and improve your well-being.

This book focuses on taking your body through movements you can easily incorporate into your daily life. This will start the process of unsticking your muscles and making them more pliable and responsive. It will also bring more movement into your spine and the other joints of your upper body, keeping everything functioning more freely and helping you to feel more energised.

Annie's story

Annie is a client whose shoulder arthritis had become so painful that it was limiting her work and home life, to the extent that surgery had been scheduled by the time she came to see us.

Using a pole, we showed Annie how to do a number of shoulder exercises and self-massages, which she found both relieving and nurturing and performed morning and evening. Within a few weeks the pain in her arthritic shoulder was much reduced. The pole work cannot cure arthritis, but it can take away tightness and pressure around it, helping the shoulder to function better. Despite the arthritis, she was now able to move without pain.

Some weeks after introducing pole work into her day, Annie triumphantly announced, 'I've cancelled my surgery as my shoulder doesn't hurt any more. I am sleeping better and I can manage everything I need to do as long as I do a few minutes a day of shoulder exercises, stretching and massage. My surgeon is amazed and he joked that he needs to use the method too, as surgery is demanding on his shoulders.'

2 WHY MODERN LIVING IS A STRAIN

We have had so many patients come to us because their neck has suddenly 'locked up' or they felt their 'shoulder go' while doing something simple, like brushing their teeth or reaching for an item in the dishwasher. However, what many people don't realise is that these simple movements weren't the cause of the problem – they were just the last straw! The underlying issue had almost certainly been present for some time until eventually a minor incident caused sudden, acute pain. That's why, in order to prevent unnecessary aches and pains, we all need to unstick our muscles and joints on a daily basis by moving our bodies in the correct way.

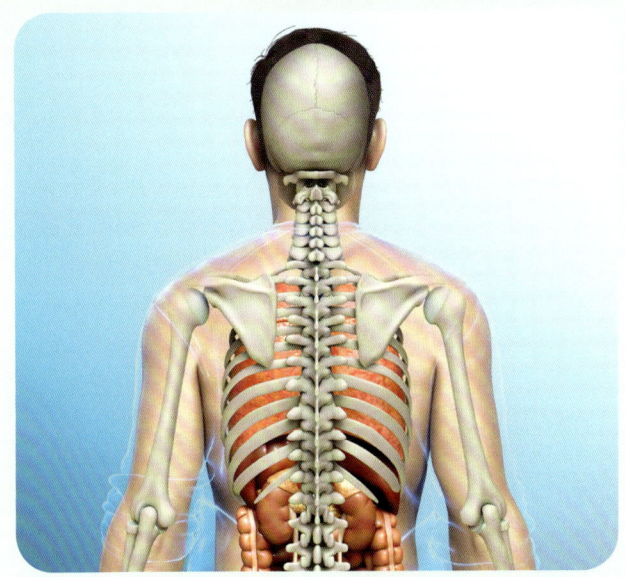

Ben's story

Ben was a typical eight-year-old boy, full of energy, who loved gaming. His parents normally limited him to an hour a day on the computer, except on special occasions. At Christmas Ben was thrilled to receive a number of exciting new games. In January he was off school for a week with a virus. While he was ill he was allowed to play his games for many more hours a day than normal.

A week later Ben woke up one morning with a painful and locked neck. His parents took him to see a doctor and various other medical practitioners and subsequently he had X-rays and scans, but nothing untoward was found. While his symptoms eased a little over time they still persisted, so two months later Ben was brought to see Andy for a thorough examination. Andy established that the real issue was that Ben's upper back, between his shoulder blades, had become so stiff that his neck had strained and gone into spasm. This was caused from having a forward head posture when gaming.

After a treatment session and two days of prescribed therapeutic exercises, Ben was pain-free by the third day. The importance of good posture and keeping his ears over his shoulders, especially when gaming, were emphasised. He was also advised to do upper back rotation exercises every day. Ben was happy to feel like a bouncy eight-year-old again and announced with a big grin that, 'It should be "movement is magic", not "movement is medicine"!'

The problem is that modern lifestyles tend to be sedentary. We spend more time sitting and less time being physically active. This has been made worse by the significant rise in remote working in recent years, often without good ergonomic set-ups. We constantly use phones, tablets and computers, which means we tend to slump forwards, rounding our upper backs and shoulders and sticking our necks out. We're all beginning to look like frozen prawns that need defrosting and uncurling! Jokes aside, looking like a prawn may not be a problem, but the discomfort and health issues that accompany poor posture are.

WEIGHING UP THE PHYSICAL DAMAGE

Next time you're in a cafe or on a train, observe people on their phones. You will spot a lot of jutting chins and 'tech neck' (the technical term for this is 'forward head posture'). Yet most people are totally unaware they are adopting this position. When using our phones we drop our heads forwards, as if the screen is a magnet drawing us towards it, and we hold our arms down and forwards. When your head protrudes forwards from your chest and shoulders in this way, it strains the muscles of your neck and upper back. The reason for this is that every 2.5cm (1in) your head sticks out, your neck and upper back must support roughly 4.5kg (10lb) of extra weight. This increases the stress on your neck and the risk of headaches, muscle imbalances and pain. Simply raising your phone to eye level, drawing your head back and resting your elbow on a support makes a huge difference.

While work and education tend to involve sitting at a desk, we spend a lot of our other time seated, too. There are a multitude of TV and streaming options on offer, so it's not surprising that the average person spends over 20 hours per week of leisure time in front of screens. To make matters worse, driving has largely replaced walking for many, and of course this involves yet more sitting. Even when we are

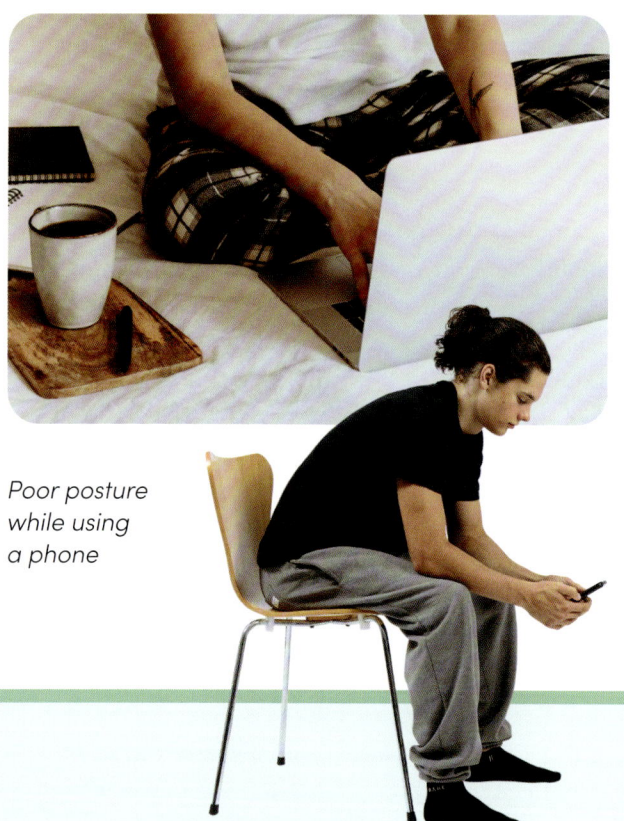

Poor posture while using a phone

active, some of the actions of daily life can have an adverse effect on the body. For instance, although gardening is certainly an active leisure pursuit, long periods spent bent forwards, perhaps weeding or planting, can put strain on the body.

Other factors play their part, too. Schoolchildren and adults often carry bags that are too heavy. The advice is that bags should weigh no more than 10 per cent of a person's body weight in order to reduce the risk of musculoskeletal problems, yet many people regularly exceed this.

The type of bag and how it is worn is also a problem. Bags should be carried on both shoulders equally or held in front with both arms, yet many young people carry backpacks on one shoulder. This loads the spine unevenly and can easily cause back or neck pain. This also applies to people carrying heavy shopping bags on one shoulder or in one hand.

Excess weight and body fat is another factor. A large belly can cause back pain, since the excess weight hangs off the spine and causes the spinal muscles to tighten up, contributing to back stiffness. Your spine is designed to move as a balanced unit and should work in a co-ordinated and flexible way. Discomfort and damage can occur if any part of your spine works in isolation while the other areas are stiff.

In addition to these external factors, the amount of movement you do can have a direct impact on the strength and mobility of your muscle tissues. Movement influences our cells, particularly those involved with maintaining structural tissues, such as our muscles. The mechanical stimulus of movement pulling on the cells encourages them to make more proteins and arrange them in such a way as to make our tissues stronger and more elastic. Unfortunately, the opposite is also true: lack of movement and the resultant lack of cell stimulus leads to weaker and stiffer tissues.

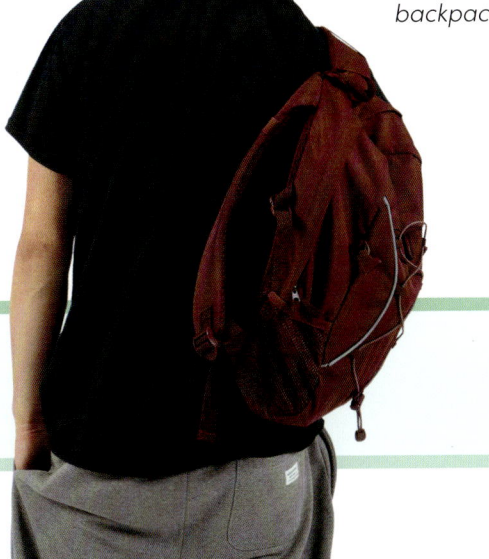

How not to carry a backpack

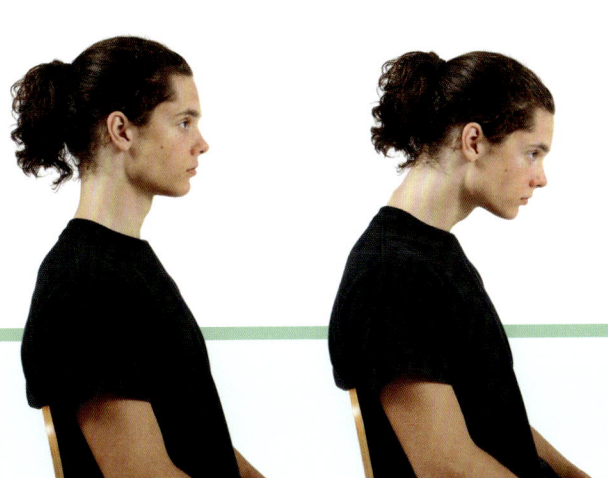

Good versus poor seated posture

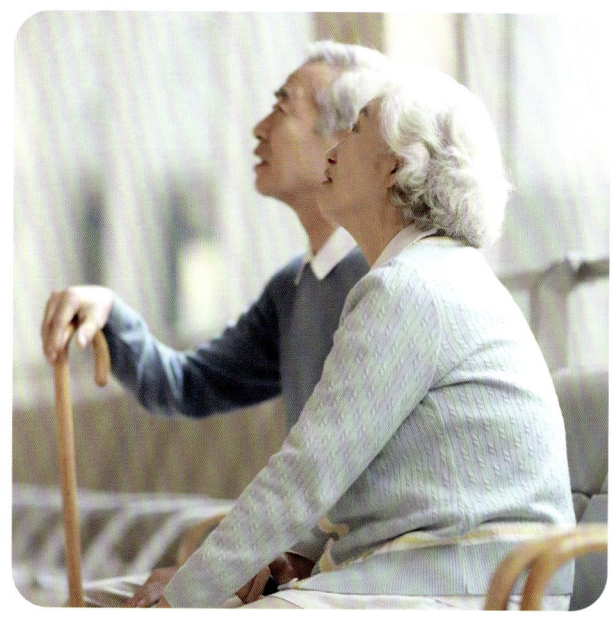

THE EFFECTS OF AGEING

From about the age of 30 we naturally lose about 1 per cent of our physiological abilities every year. Then from 60 onwards our natural loss of muscle mass and strength starts to speed up. We can counteract this, though, with regular and varied exercises. Resistance training in particular is important to help maintain strong and healthy muscles, and keeping your joints and muscles mobile helps make resistance training easier, enabling muscular strength to be used properly.

Some people believe that as we reach our senior years stooping is inevitable. However, this isn't the case, because with the correct actions you can maintain an elegant upright posture as you age. If you persistently round your shoulders and hunch your upper back (the medical term for this is 'kyphosis') then that position will become normal for you, and it will be difficult and painful to change it. If you act now, you can potentially avoid it and the earlier you take action the easier it is to prevent rounding and hunching. It is good to know that positive changes can be made at any age.

We all know that if we repeatedly bend a stick at one point, it will end up breaking. The same principle applies to your spine: if you keep bending or hinging it at only one point it is likely to become damaged. We need to keep the whole spine mobile with all its parts working together. This is particularly worth remembering when you are gardening or enjoying other leisure activities.

The good news is that it is easy to look after your joints and muscles when you know how, but however old – or young – you are, you need to keep them moving. If you wake a hibernating bear you would expect it to be a bit grizzly. Dormant muscles are the same. Keep them awake and active, and they won't complain by aching, although if your muscles do go into hibernation it's never too late to wake them and get them going again.

'Gentle' and 'easing into' are two important approaches to keep in mind as you try the movements in this book, especially if you are older. They are all safe, but by doing them in a controlled manner you'll ensure that you get the maximum benefit. As you get used to a movement or stretch, your range of pain-free movement should increase.

DEALING WITH PAIN

Your upper back, neck and shoulders need to work smoothly together as a team, and if you have pain in a particular part of your upper body it is often because other associated areas

ACTIVE PAIN RELIEF

Research has shown that using either a hot or a cold pack for pain relief works equally well because both distract the brain from the pain and they are a good alternative to pain medication.

However, you should avoid using hot or cold therapy in areas of poor circulation, or reduced sensation. You should also ensure that the hot or cold pack is not too extreme and is wrapped in a tea towel or similar, to avoid skin burn.

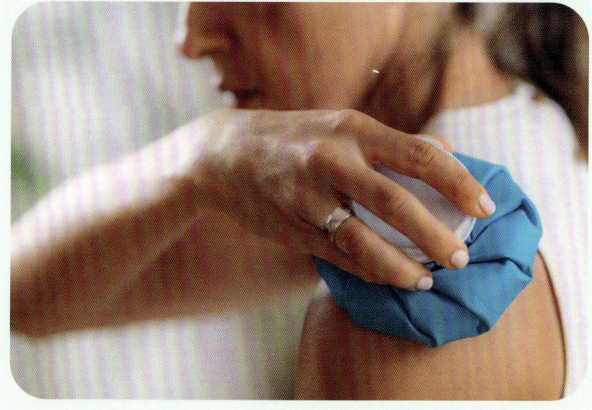

If you have a sharp pain from injuring yourself, or if you are aching and need pain relief, trying the following can be useful:

- Apply a wrapped cold pack to the area as soon as possible and hold it there for at least 15 minutes. (The minimum application time required for a hot or cold pack to produce effective local pain relief is 15 minutes.)
- If the cold pack does not feel right for you, try a heat pack for 15 minutes.
- Or try alternating hot and cold packs for 5 minutes each, for a total of 20 minutes. This hot and cold pattern can increase the effectiveness of the relief.
- The sessions of hot/cold packs can be repeated 3–4 times a day but allow at least an hour for the area to cool down or warm up in between the sessions.
- After applying the hot or cold pack for 15 minutes, gently rub the area for 30 seconds or so, to help restore normal blood flow.
- When the issue is more of an ache in the muscles, a hot pack can often be more effective.

are not moving well. The tightness tests (see pp. 42–53) will help you identify which areas in your upper body are tight and need attention. By acting on the results of your tests, you can prioritise the most important areas to work on. For example, if your shoulder hurts but the tests say you're stiff in your upper back, then you will know that rather than just doing shoulder exercises and self-massages, you also need to do regular upper back work.

Working towards pain, but stopping before you experience it, is helpful because it can improve your upper body comfort and mobility by increasing your circulation and range of movement and reducing your tightness. However, you should never ignore, try to push through or work with pain, as this can damage your muscles and joints. That would then be counterproductive, since you would need to rest to allow the tissues to recover.

PAIN-FREE MOVEMENT

Everyone is different and symptoms of pain, discomfort, aching, stiffness and restricted movement in the upper body can vary greatly. Regardless of whether you are able to walk or stand comfortably, or have general aches or specific points of pain, there are exercises and self-massages in this book that will help you, but the key is to first start and then to continue taking small steps on your journey to becoming physically comfortable.

We all need to move, even a little bit, every hour of the day. Interestingly, we tend to move naturally every 15 minutes or so, even when we're asleep, as our bodies instinctively try to prevent a build-up of stiffness in our joints and muscles. That's why it's better to do a little and often rather than a lot occasionally, even if your movements are mini or even micro, but it also helps if you know how to perform a simple movement like looking down without putting stresses and strains on your body.

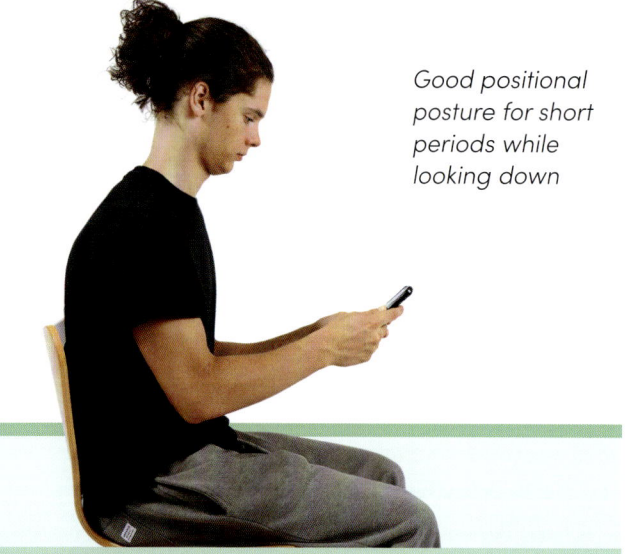

Good positional posture for short periods while looking down

Nim's story

Nim was a sporty 22-year-old who worked full time, sitting at a computer in an office. In her lunch breaks she often took a brisk walk and in the evenings she played netball or tennis or went to the gym.

One weekend she was in a pub with her friend, waiting at the bar. When she went to order, searing pain radiated down one side of her neck and into her back. She tried to catch her breath and move her neck, but the pain remained.

In her final year at school Nim had worked as a Saturday receptionist for Andy. She now called him, and he explained that spending all day at her computer had caused her back to get tight and stiff. What she needed was to move her whole upper spine in a balanced way while working at her computer, so one part of her spine would not become repeatedly overworked.

Andy estimated it might take a week for her neck to settle, and that in the meantime she would need to use heat and cold packs and pain medication. He also sent her videos of seated exercises that she could do to help herself.

It took four days for Nim's neck to recover, but the experience motivated her to do desk exercises regularly. Her colleagues now join her in taking movement medicine breaks.

How to look down for a short time

Having your head and neck in a forward position for long periods damages your body, so this is how to look down for a relatively short time at something close to you – for example, a plate of food or your shoes – using your whole spine:

WHY MODERN LIVING IS A STRAIN

- Stand or sit in neutral posture (*see* p. 35 or p. 38), upright with your shoulders gently drawn back and your ears over your shoulders.
- To look at something close to you for a short time, allow your whole spine to curve forwards as you start to look down, while trying to keep your ears in line with your shoulders.
- To support your spine and prevent yourself from collapsing forwards, pull in your tummy muscles (the core muscles that wrap around your lower trunk and support your lower back and pelvis). To help, place one hand at the top of your tummy, just below your chest bone and one below your tummy button.
- Gently pull in through the muscles under your hands and allow your whole spine, including your neck, to curve forwards as you start to look down. Think of your spine lengthening up and over as you do so and keep your shoulders drawn back and down.
- At the same time, try to keep your head drawn gently back, so your ears stay in line with your shoulders and your head isn't dropped or thrust forwards.
- After looking down for a few moments, return to a good upright posture again.

How to look down for longer

Sometimes, of course, you need to look forwards and down at something that is slightly further away and for a longer period of time, for example, when you're looking at some papers in the middle of a large table or sitting up in the stands of a stadium watching a match. Ideally, you should be standing or sitting in an upright neutral posture so all you have to do to follow proceedings is adjust your eyes or head slightly, but if that isn't possible then the following advice will help:

- Start by standing or sitting tall in an upright neutral posture (*see* p. 35 or p. 38) with your tummy gently pulled in.
- If you're sitting at a table, maintain length through your spine and lean forwards from the hips, keeping your ears in line with your shoulders, and rest your arms on the table. Keep your shoulders down (the technical term is 'placed') and lean some weight on your arms.
- If there is nothing to lean on, interlace your fingers, keep your shoulders placed and lean your forearms on your thighs. Better still, try to position something on your lap and lean on that. Be sure to keep lengthened through your spine and to keep your head drawn back, so that your ears are in line with your shoulders.
- As often as you can, return to an upright neutral posture and if possible walk around or do some neck settling movements (*see* p. 81).

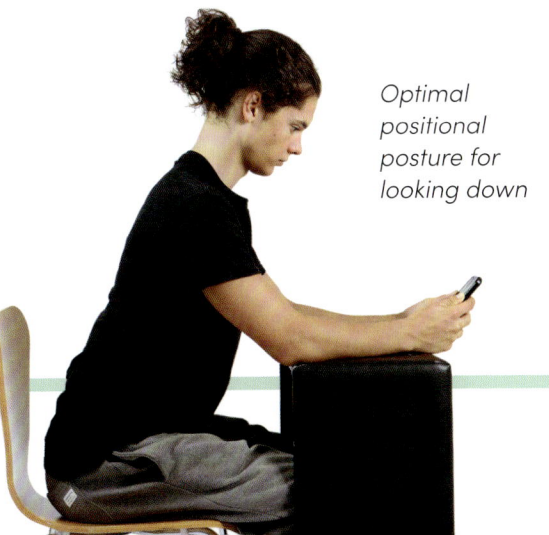

Optimal positional posture for looking down

3 UNDERSTANDING HOW YOUR BODY MOVES

The structures of your body that are involved in movement are quite complicated, so in an effort to provide an easier understanding, consider the following simplified picture. Lying beneath the skin layer of your body lies your fascia, a bodysuit covering and surrounding the muscles, bones and internal organs. This helps to give the body shape. The fascia also joins your muscles to your bones and the muscles to each other, enabling your muscles to contract and produce movement by pulling on the bones and other muscles.

Fascia is organised in layers and has lots of water in it. This helps different muscles to glide over each other and also for muscles to glide over bones without causing soreness.

Your fascia covers everything, even your head, hands and feet, providing cushioning and protection, and helps stabilise your joints by keeping your bones aligned and preventing them dislocating or moving too much.

Away from your joints, your fascia moves more freely, allowing your body a full range of movement. You can feel these differences yourself if you compare the looseness of the tissues in the middle of your upper arm or thigh with the relative tightness of the tissues around your elbow or knee.

However, if you remain inactive for long periods, or have an injury or surgery and don't rehabilitate properly, your fascia can stop working so well. The different layers should slide smoothly over each other, but instead they can get stuck to each other, which can cause aching or stiffness.

What's more, a restriction in one area can generate problems further away by making those areas overcompensate and take too much strain. For example, restrictions in your upper back may cause pain and dysfunction in your neck or shoulder, or a strain in your neck or shoulder could result from limited movement in fascia that is tight or twisted around your chest.

Your fascia is living tissue, so it is always adjusting its shape and length according to your posture and movements. If you sit slumped forwards for long periods, the fascia on your chest and the front of your ribcage will shorten. This then makes it much harder to sit upright and can give you a hunched upper back. Happily, paying attention to your posture (*see* pp. 34–40) and doing the exercises and self-massages we recommend can help.

WHY MOVEMENT IS ESSENTIAL

To keep your body's fascia functioning smoothly it's essential to engage in regular movement and exercise, as we've seen. This also helps to rebalance your fascia, which is particularly important if your work or leisure posture has created asymmetries. Provided that you are taking in sufficient water and nutrients, movement helps your body deliver them to where they are needed most. This includes delivering them to the fascia.

The communication between your brain and your body is a two-way process. Messages go

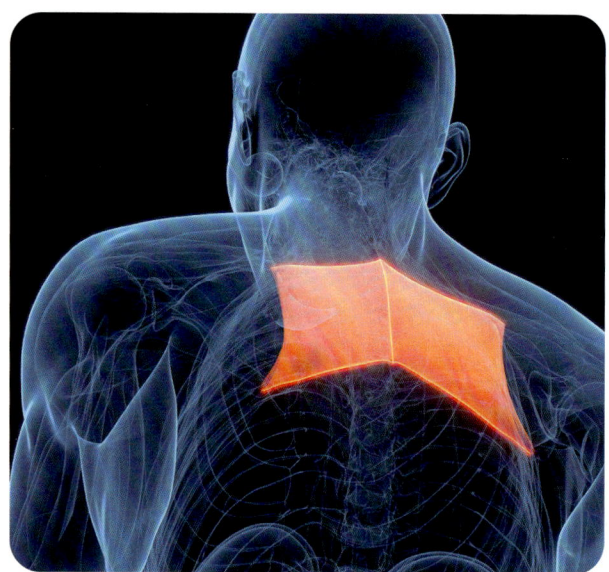

Diagram of the upper back/thorax

upright posture when you're at rest, your body will respond according to your instructions and rebuild to a healthy shape.

HOW YOUR UPPER BACK WORKS

In this book we focus on the upper back, neck and shoulders. When we refer to your 'upper back', we are including the spine (from the base of the neck to the bottom of your ribs), ribs and chest, medically known as your thorax. This acts as a protective shield for vital organs such as the heart, lungs and spinal cord.

Your upper back also plays a crucial role in maintaining good posture, because when kept healthy it enables you to maintain an upright and balanced stance and provides support for your head, neck and shoulders.

Flexibility in your upper back is important for lots of reasons. For example, when you're cycling or driving and stop at a junction, you need to look each way before proceeding. You might not think this involves your upper back, but as you turn your head and neck, there needs to be sufficient flexibility in your upper back to allow it to turn slightly too, to reduce the risk of neck strain.

Your upper back also has an important role in the co-ordination and control of movements such as walking, running and climbing. For example, when you're walking, for co-ordinated arm and leg movements to happen smoothly there needs to be a slight rotation through your upper back, with each rotation storing some energy to help power the next stride. The soft tissues linking your arms and legs pass over and through your upper back and they need to be able to glide a little as you move. If your upper

from the brain to the body to initiate movement. The fascia, which is richly supplied with nerve endings, is the main tissue that sends sensory feedback to the spinal cord and brain, informing them of the body's position and the forces that are acting on it. Regular movement keeps this communication loop healthy and functioning well.

The body's blood vessels, lymph vessels and nerves also require movement to function optimally. Without it they can become sluggish or even trapped.

Our bodies are continually being renewed, and how your muscles and fascia are remodelled depends on the instructions and directions you give them through your movements and posture. If you stay hunched for prolonged periods without movement breaks, your body will rebuild using the information that a stiff, hunched position is the shape you want it to take. If you regularly return to an back is stiff, it can't rotate and the tissues can't glide across each other easily, which makes walking more energy-consuming and also increases the risk of injury.

Flexibility is also important so that the upper back can act as a shock absorber. Imagine walking towards a door and going to push it open with your outstretched arm but finding that the door is heavier than you thought. If your upper back is too stiff and unable to absorb some of the shock, then you are more likely to injure your shoulder, neck, arm or even your upper back itself when opening the door.

How to keep your upper back healthy

When you're sitting down during the day, or even standing around for long periods, to keep your upper back healthy you need to move, stretch and self-massage for at least a few minutes every hour. You also need to maintain good posture (see Chapter 4) to avoid getting aches and pains from sitting or standing with a hunched upper back.

Part of being able to maintain good posture is moving frequently and gently, so that your nerves can sense what position your body is in. Without movement, these nerves can switch off, leaving you unaware of how you are sitting or standing.

Easy, efficient breathing is also essential to good health, but to do this requires your diaphragm, ribs and upper back to allow air to move easily in and out of your lungs. If your upper back is stiff from lack of movement, it can make breathing more difficult. This, in turn, can leave you feeling more tired and stressed, as well as increasing the likelihood of neck, shoulder and back aches and a hunched posture. It can also make you more prone to respiratory infections.

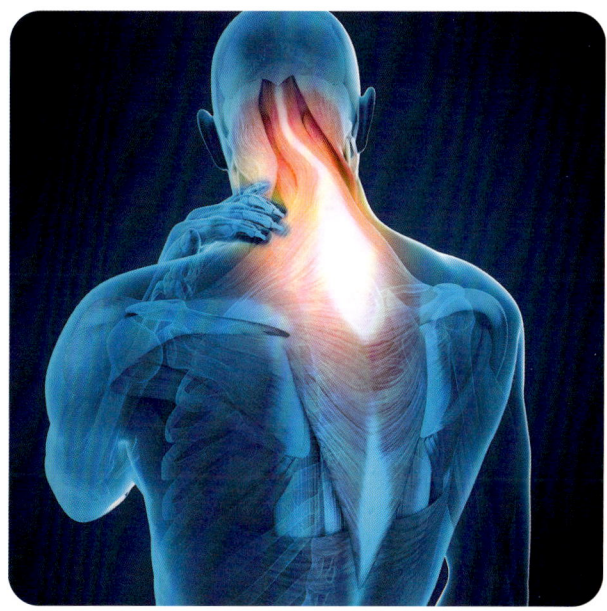

Diagram of the neck

HOW YOUR NECK WORKS

The neck has several crucial functions. It supports the weight of your head, allows you to turn, nod and tilt your head, and keeps your head level and balanced. It also acts as a shock absorber, protecting your brain from injury, especially if you fall. When your neck becomes painful you soon notice that everyday activities become difficult.

At the centre of the neck is the cervical spine, a stack of seven neck bones that form a strong yet flexible column to support the head, protect the spinal cord and facilitate movement. Between these neck bones are discs made of cartilage, which help keep the bones aligned, provide cushioning and allow for gentle twisting. At the back of the neck are the facet joints, which help to control and provide stability for neck movement. The facet joints also help to distribute the various forces that act on the spine when you sit, stand, walk or lift something. By sharing this load with the discs, muscles and ligaments, stress is distributed along the spine. The long ligaments in the neck act like support stockings and work together with the discs to keep the neck bones stable, but mobile.

How to keep your neck healthy

To keep your neck healthy you need to avoid staying in one position for too long; as with the other parts of your body, you need to move your neck a little and often. Daily stretching will also help keep your neck muscles lengthened and responsive. If you self-massage tight and restricted neck muscles you will release tension that can easily build up during the day, particularly when working at a computer or desk.

Combining movement, stretching and self-massage is the most effective way of keeping your neck healthy, because together they increase blood flow, reduce stiffness and maintain mobility. This will improve your neck's function and prevent pain and headaches. Without including these activities in your daily routine, it is very difficult to maintain the good posture (*see* Chapter 4) that will enable your neck to remain relaxed.

HOW YOUR SHOULDERS WORK

Healthy shoulders that function well are essential for carrying out the many tasks we do as humans, from hugging loved ones, to doing up a bra or a zip on your back, to getting something down from the top shelf. The functionality of our shoulders is also crucial to helping our hands do what we need them to.

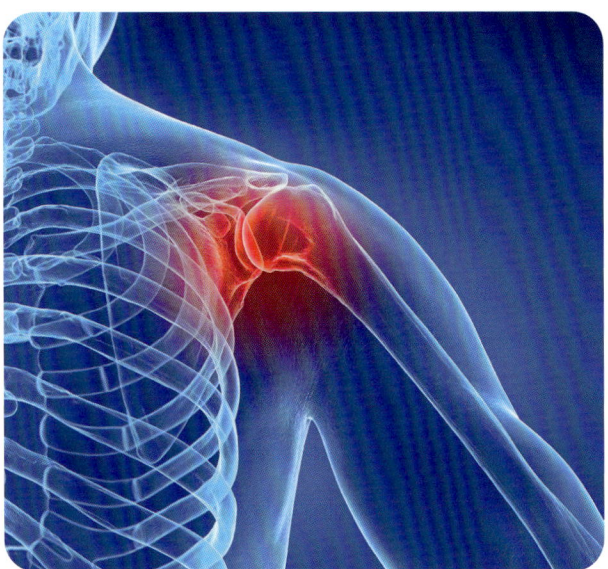

Diagram of the shoulder

The shoulder is one of the most complicated joints in our bodies. It has two main parts. One is a ball-and-socket joint, which consists of the round head of the upper arm bone and the relatively shallow socket on the outside of the shoulder blade. The other is a joint between the shoulder blade and ribs, which enables the shoulder blade to glide over the ribs. This allows you to lift, throw and reach in many directions.

Wrapped around the ball and socket joint is the rotator cuff, a collection of muscles and tendons that hold the shoulder joint in place. The rotator cuff helps reduce the risk of shoulder injury while allowing the joint to move through its maximum range. During any arm and shoulder movement the rotator cuff continuously adjusts the tension of its different parts to make the movement as smooth as possible. While the muscles in your rotator cuff are good at controlling the movement of your ball-and-socket joint, they are not well-suited to providing the power required to move your arm. This comes from your shoulder's larger muscles, which run from your upper body to your arm bone.

How to keep your shoulders healthy

To maintain healthy shoulder function and protect our shoulders from accidental damage we need to keep them supple. We can achieve that by regularly taking the shoulder joints and rotator cuff muscles through their full range of movements. With modern living, this often doesn't happen, as we do almost all our daily activities with our arms down and forwards. This can cause pain and restricted movement to develop in your shoulder. Luckily, you can address this if you carry out appropriate exercises (*see* Chapter 8).

While repetitive strain or injury can certainly cause shoulder issues, in our experience if you're not looking after your shoulder joints, muscles and tissues with regular movements, stretches and self-massages then you are at greater risk of injuring yourself. If your shoulders are not conditioned and evenly balanced and you sustain an injury, it will also take longer to recover.

> **THE BENEFITS OF ASSISTED HANGING FOR THE SHOULDERS**
>
> Hanging stretches help keep the shoulder joint open, as well as maintaining healthy and balanced shoulder, upper back and arm muscles.
>
> However, when people talk of hanging in relation to the shoulders they are usually referring to hanging straight down from both arms with both feet off the floor. This is not how our shoulders are designed to work, though. When we climb a tree or a ladder we reach up with one arm at a time, so that arm can take the weight, which is why we have taken the concept of hanging and made it multidirectional and easier on the body by introducing a pole.

4 HOW TO ACHIEVE GOOD POSTURE

Good posture promotes health and a feeling of strength and vitality. Standing upright with an open chest and relaxed shoulders can immediately make you feel more confident. A neutral and natural posture is perfectly balanced, and is the golden key to feeling, functioning and moving well.

Slouching places excessive and unnecessary stress on your spine, muscles and discs, and compresses your nerves and joints. Hunching your back and rounding your shoulders causes upper back, neck and shoulder pain, and limits your body's ability to function freely. Poor posture can also result in headaches, reduced concentration, aches, muscle knots and tiredness.

Knowing what good posture is and then prioritising and maintaining it is vital if you want your body to work well. Good posture allows your lungs to expand as much as possible, maximising the intake of oxygen and the removal of carbon dioxide, and improving your respiratory function. This supports your circulation and ensures your bodily tissues stay healthy. Even your brain, core and pelvic floor work better when you maintain a neutral posture.

If you're a sports or fitness enthusiast, good posture enables you to perform at your best, with the muscles throughout your body working in balance, maximising the full range of motion. Good posture also improves agility and co-ordination, helps prevent falls, and optimises your digestion and breathing.

NEUTRAL POSTURE

Neutral posture refers to the natural position of the body, and a way of standing or sitting that puts the least amount of strain on your upper back, neck and shoulders. A neutral posture is particularly important if you're carrying out demanding physical tasks, such as lifting heavy items. As a reminder of the importance of neutral posture, in Part 2 we often ask you to start in neutral.

How to achieve neutral posture in standing

Good posture is not meant to be a fixed or permanent position, but it's the healthiest one to work from and to return to whenever possible. We have provided some simple step-by-step tips to help you positively adjust your posture in standing, focusing on one area at a time. This will help you gain a thorough understanding and create the muscle memory for how to position your body correctly.

We suggest you initially work against a wall and, if you can, in front of a mirror, so you can get instant physical and visual feedback. However, having used the wall to help you gain good posture, move away from it and try to maintain the same posture.

Franco's story

Franco is a highly skilled specialist dental surgeon. He deals with complex cases and spends many hours a day in surgery, which requires the most advanced skills, extremely steady hands and excellent concentration.

Naturally this close-up work means that he leans forward for many hours and also works with his arms unsupported. He was exercising daily but had not realised that his posture needed a slight correction. He did not appear round shouldered or particularly hunched, but he did have a forward head posture. As this had become his norm he was beginning to experience stabbing pain in the neck and in his upper back just below one shoulder blade. When he did surgery, he was able to block it out, but it was becoming so bad that it was making it difficult for him to sleep or drive.

We encouraged Franco to focus on having his ears in line with his shoulders as much as possible when in surgery and without question the rest of the time, especially when driving.

Franco was already doing the three essential upper back moves (*see* p. 116) each evening but now added in self-massage and stretching to his back and neck. He found these very relieving and a pleasure to do and together with the conscious postural adjustments they helped to take away his stabbing pain.

1. Get into position

- Stand with your back against a wall. Place your feet hip-width apart and 10–20cm (4–8in) away from the wall. Your buttocks, upper back and shoulder blades should be touching the wall. Your head should be able to lightly touch the wall and your ears should be over your shoulders with your chin level. (If you find it hard to get the back of your head to touch the wall then place a small cushion behind your head.)
- Stand with even pressure through both feet.
- Your legs should be straight. Don't bend at the knee, but don't push your knees backwards either, as this will overextend them. Your hips should be square and level and not twisted.
- There should be a small curve in your lower back and behind the back of your neck, giving a natural slight space between your lower back and neck and the wall.

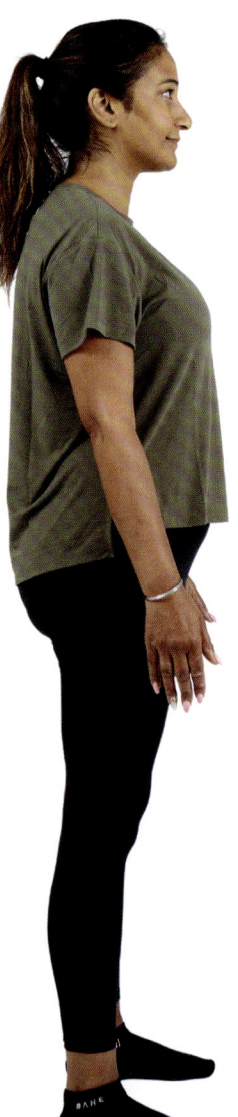

Neutral posture in standing

2. Lengthen your spine

- Make yourself taller by lengthening yourself upwards through the top of your spine and downwards through the bottom of your spine.
- It may help to imagine a dot in the middle of your chest bone and a dot on your upper back, just below your neck. Try to lift the two dots up as high as you can; this will be a subtle rather than a massive movement.
- You can think of a third dot on your tailbone and you gently lengthen it down.

3. Draw your head and neck back

- Lengthen through your upper back and spine. Imagine two helium balloons are attached to the bones just behind your ears, one on each side, and they are gently lifting the back of the head.
- Now ease the back of your head towards the wall behind, but don't force it.
- Keep your chin level with the floor and look ahead as you try to have your ears over the middle of your shoulders, rather than in front of them.

4. Relax your shoulders

- Let your arms lengthen by your sides with the palms facing forwards.
- Lift your shoulders towards your ears and release them by sliding your shoulder blades towards your back pockets. Try to let the front of your shoulders open towards the sides of the room as your shoulder blades at the back draw towards each other a little.
- Pause for a few moments and feel your muscles gently working around the back of your underarms, shoulders and shoulder blades.
- Let your arms relax by your sides and your palms turn in towards your thighs. Imagine you are holding a baguette under each arm. This encourages your muscles to remain working gently, while keeping your shoulders in place and supported.

5. Relax your ribs down

- Keeping your tummy in, take a big breath and then let out a big sigh to allow your ribs to relax, but don't push them down or out, because that creates tension in your shoulders or upper back. Once your ribs are relaxed, breathe normally.

6. Pull your tummy in

- Gently pull in your tummy muscles (the core muscles that wrap around your lower trunk and support your lower back and pelvis) towards your spine, and then add a gentle uplift. Think 'in scoop, up scoop'. This is a similar feeling to pulling your tummy in to do up a zip on a tight pair of trousers, sucking in equally above and below your belly button.

7. Tighten your buttocks

- Imagine you have two magnets attached to the top of each of your inner thighs and that they are being drawn towards each other. Then imagine the same magnets are also being pulled and drawn towards another magnet, which is positioned in your lower abdomen. You will notice your buttocks tighten slightly to support your back.

8. Tighten your pelvic floor

- The magnet visualisation helps your pelvic floor muscles to work, but you can also gently tighten them by imagining trying to stop a wee and wind at the same time. The aim is to get a feeling of lifting the pelvic floor. It may help to think about your pelvic floor muscles as a band running from your pubic bone to your tailbone (front to back). Another band runs between your two sit bones/bottom bones (side to side). If you mentally join these points up it creates the diamond shape of your pelvic floor area.

How to achieve neutral posture in sitting

Below are some simple step-by-step tips to help you positively adjust your posture when sitting. Remember that posture adjustments should not be forced: they should be eased into. Posture should be viewed as 'fluid'.

1. Get into position

- Sit on a chair that positions you so that your hips are at the same or a slightly higher level than your knees.
- Your feet should be hip-width apart and under or slightly in front of your knees.
- There should be equal pressure on each buttock.
- If you're working at a desk, your forearms and wrists need to be supported and your screen should be at eye level.
- It is essential that the upper back has some elasticity in order for the rest of the body to be properly aligned. It can be difficult to align the head, neck and shoulders into good posture if the upper back and ribs are stiff or rounding, so relax these areas.

2. Now perform steps 2 to 6 as outlined in 'How achieve neutral posture in standing' (*see* pp. 36–7).

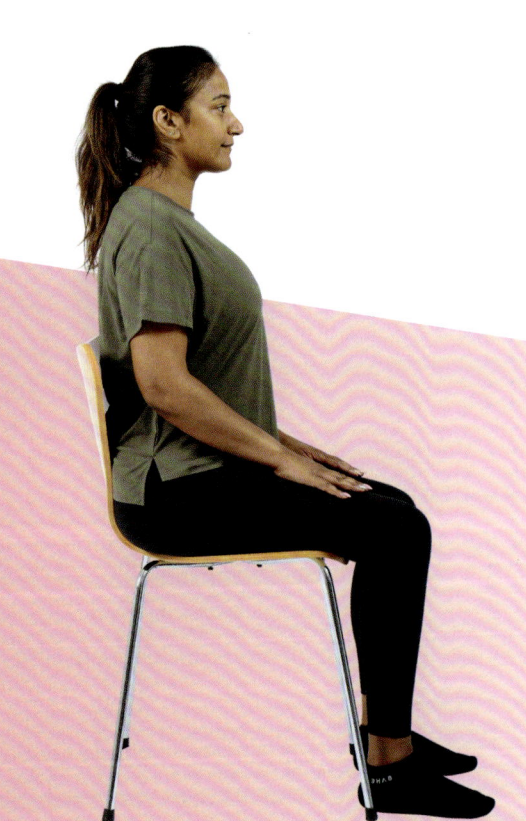

Neutral posture in sitting

HOW TO BREATHE

Breathing and good posture are intimately related. Maintaining good posture helps you breathe more easily and healthy breathing helps you maintain good posture. When both are optimised, you will experience fewer upper body aches and pains, your body will work more effectively and you'll have a greater sense of well-being.

As you breathe, try to keep your tummy gently pulled in towards your spine. When you breathe out, imagine that you are gently blowing a candle flame to make it flicker. When exercising, you should ideally breathe in through your nose and out through your mouth. Breathing in through your nose releases nitric oxide into your airways, which helps expand them and the blood vessels in your lungs and improves oxygen uptake. Nose-breathing also helps filter impurities and humidifies the air, both of which are better for the lungs.

It is very common to forget to breathe when concentrating on an exercise. We say 'blow to go' to help people remember to blow their breath out as they start a movement and then to breathe in through the nose. This ensures you don't hold your breath, which increases internal pressure and unwanted tension.

How to perform 'smiley' breathing

We also use a technique called 'smiley' breathing to help the lower ribs open for deeper and healthier breathing. The lungs are pear-shaped, so more air enters them if you breathe into your lower ribcage. Smiley breathing also helps improve movement in the upper back, where your ribs join your spine, which reduces stiffness and makes the upper back more pliable for improved movement. A ribcage that has good elasticity also recoils naturally, making breathing out easier.

Good breathing follows if you have a relaxed, open and upright neutral posture. If you slump, your upper back and ribs become less elastic and your breathing becomes restricted and more difficult.

- Stand or sit in an upright neutral posture (*see* p. 35 or p. 38). Keep your ears over your shoulders and your shoulders down. Place your hands over your lower ribs and gently pull in your tummy.

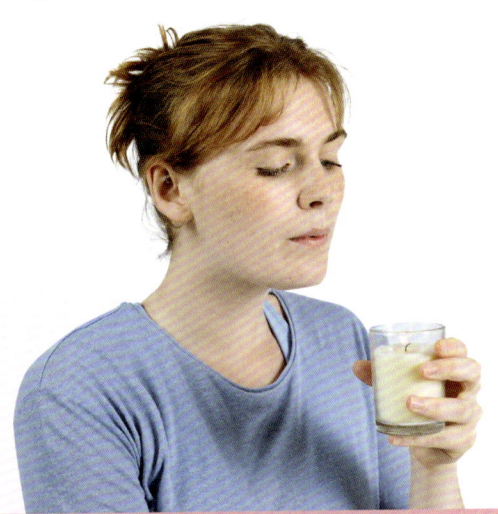

Example of blowing a candle flame to make it flicker

- Take a slow, deep breath in through your nose, keeping your tummy in. As you feel your lower ribs begin to move outwards, allow your mouth to smile widely and think of your lower ribs opening into a big smile, too.
- Continue breathing in until you reach a comfortable end point, holding your breath for a couple of seconds and keeping your shoulders down.
- Purse your lips to slowly blow your breath out. You will feel your ribs start to lower and come towards each other again.
- Continue breathing out until you reach a comfortable end point. Hold for a couple of seconds again before relaxing into the start position.
- Repeat this exercise two or three times, taking as big a breath as you comfortably can, and then return to your normal breathing pattern.

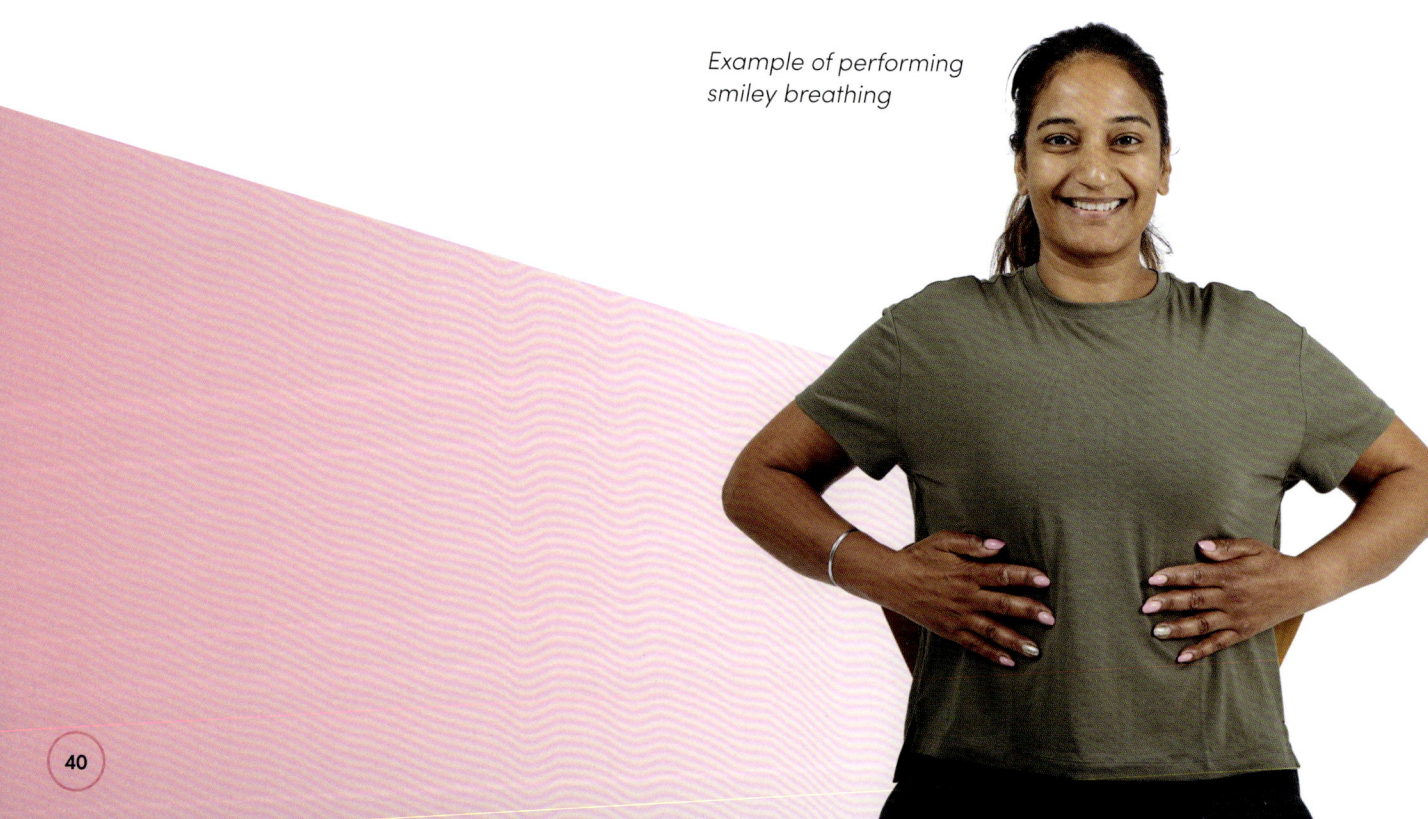

Example of performing smiley breathing

5 TIGHTNESS TESTS

Different people have different ranges of movement and what might be normal for one person may not be normal for someone else. However, so that you can gain an insight into the general flexibility and range of movement of your own upper back, neck and shoulders we have devised some simple tests. We have also suggested some stretches to get you started based on your results.

Quick and easy to carry out, these tests will really help you gain a better awareness of your body. By scoring yourself for each test and each side of the body individually, you can use the results to help you choose which exercises and massages to do. What's more, if you jot down your results and the date, you can compare and contrast the results over time as a way of measuring your progress with the Make Movement Your Medicine method. This can be hugely rewarding and motivating.

You may already be aware of discomfort in your upper body – perhaps your neck hurts and the tests tell you that not only is your neck tight but your upper back is too. So you realise from the tests that you should concentrate on both of these areas. These tests can also reveal tightness that you are unaware of. This enables you to take steps to remedy the situation before the tightness starts to give you aches or pains.

If you do discover tightness that is restricting your normal range of movement, there are various movements, stretches and self-massages that can help. A table below each set of tests will inform you which would be most helpful for your particular area of concern.

When doing any of the following tests you may find that your mobility is more limited on one side than the other. This is very common and it is not something to worry about, but it makes sense to spend more time on exercises that work on improving the range of movement on your stiffer side.

A WORD OF CAUTION

As you do the tests, don't push yourself to a point where it becomes painful. If you are unable to even start a test without causing sharp pain, then don't do it. Instead, consult a medical professional.

Also, with all these tests, do bear in mind that everyone is different and studies have shown that even for the same person the range of movement can vary slightly depending on things such as time of day, stress levels and hydration. Remember, too, that our natural range of movement decreases as we age but we can prevent or slow this down by doing activities like those in our Make Movement Your Medicine.

Lucy's story

Lucy, a high board diver, came to us with a shoulder rotator cuff (*see* p. 32) injury. Divers require strong powerful shoulders, and after years of intensive weekly training, Lucy had developed her first rotator cuff issue.

While waiting for a shoulder scan, Lucy sought our help. The rehabilitation exercises for her shoulders, she had previously been given, were not alleviating her pain. Her upper back had become too stiff and unable to take any of the impact on entering the water. This meant that her shoulders took all the force of entering the pool and inevitably became injured and painful.

Lucy performed the tightness tests and was very surprised to realise her upper back rotation was restricted, and that this was the root cause of her shoulder problem.

We gave her a personalised exercise prescription that started with the essential upper back/spine movements daily followed by forward and side partial hanging to release her upper back and shoulder tightness. She did therapeutic movements and self-massage too. Lucy only worked in a pain-free range. She experienced a significantly greater range of pain-free movement in her injured shoulder after only a few minutes of first doing these.

Lucy continued with the Breakspear Make Movement Your Medicine method (MMYM) prescription each day at home.

At the end of two weeks she attempted some easy diving. To her delight, her shoulder was no longer painful and she felt more free and stronger in her upper back, particularly between her shoulder blades. Now Lucy's upper back was not so tight she could resume diving without damaging her shoulder again. Lucy's muscles felt slightly sore from her initial return to diving training, but she no longer experienced pain or restricted shoulder movement, as long as she did a few minutes of the MMYM daily. She cancelled her scan too!

Lucy now realises the importance of keeping her upper back mobile to enable her shoulders to work well and to avoid injury when diving. She is very happy to be able to continue with the sport she loves and is no longer fearful of being forced to retire due to unnecessary shoulder injury.

UPPER BACK STIFFNESS TEST

For this simple self-assessment you are testing how far you can turn your upper back to each side, which will give you a good idea of how flexible it is. It is easiest to assess how far you can turn if you do the tests in front of a mirror:

1. Sit upright at the front of a stable chair with space to move on either side.
2. Put your feet and knees together to keep your hips still.
3. Hold your arms straight out and interlace your fingers, pointing your index fingers forwards.
4. Relax your shoulders and keep your tummy in.
5. Breathe in and as you breathe out, smoothly turn your upper back, arms and head as far as you can to one side. It is important to keep your elbows straight.
6. Your index fingers are like a pointer on a dial and indicate how far you can turn.
7. Repeat on the other side. Note down your results and refer to table 5.1 to assess your results.

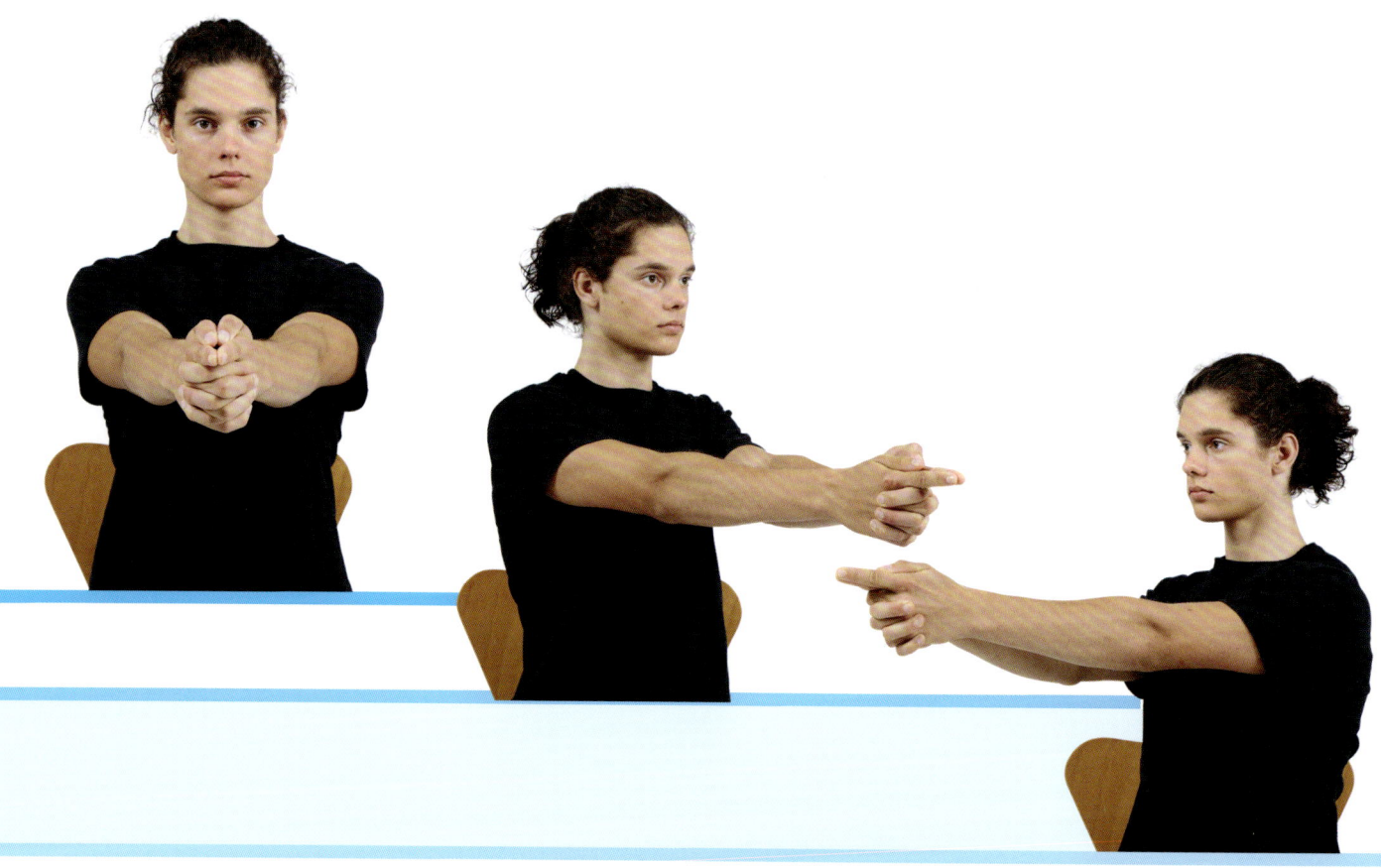

Table 5.1 Upper back mobility test results

You can easily turn beyond 45 degrees on either side	You can almost turn to 45 degrees on either side	You find it difficult to reach 45 degrees on either side
Your upper back mobility is good. To help maintain this try the Upper Back Option 1 or Option 2 sequences in table 9.2 on p. 118.	Your upper back mobility is reasonable but can be improved. Try these exercises: **1.** Two-arm swipe (*see* p. 67) **2.** Chest and shoulder release A or B (*see* pp. 72–3) **3.** Spinal muscle massage (*see* p. 74) Or try the Upper Back Option 1 or Option 2 sequences in table 9.2 on p. 118 or the Rounding Posture Option 1 or Option 2 sequences in table 9.25 on p. 164.	You will feel better if you improve your upper back mobility, so let's get started. Try these exercises: **1.** Upper back rotation, lying (*see* p. 63) **2.** One-arm forward hang, standing or seated (*see* p. 104) **3.** Upper back massage (*see* p. 75) Or try the Upper Back Option 1 or Option 2 sequences in table 9.2 on p. 118 or the Rounding Posture Option 1 or Option 2 sequences in table 9.25 on p. 164.

NECK ROTATION TEST

The neck has an amazing set of varied joints that allow for quite complicated movements. This and the following test will give you an idea of how much neck mobility you have and what you may need to work on. It is easiest to assess how far you can rotate your neck if you do the tests in front of a mirror:

1. Sit upright at the back of a stable chair.
2. Rest one hand on the middle of your upper chest, with your index finger just resting on your chin.
3. Hold your other arm straight out to the side and in line with your chest.
4. Relax your shoulders and keep your tummy in.
5. Breathe in and as you breathe out, smoothly turn your head in the direction of your outstretched arm, as far as you comfortably can without straining, keeping the rest of your upper body still and not moving your finger (as in, don't move it with your chin).
6. The angle between your finger and where your chin reaches will indicate how far you can turn, which should ideally be at least 45 degrees.
7. Repeat on the other side. Note down your results and refer to table 5.2 to assess your results.

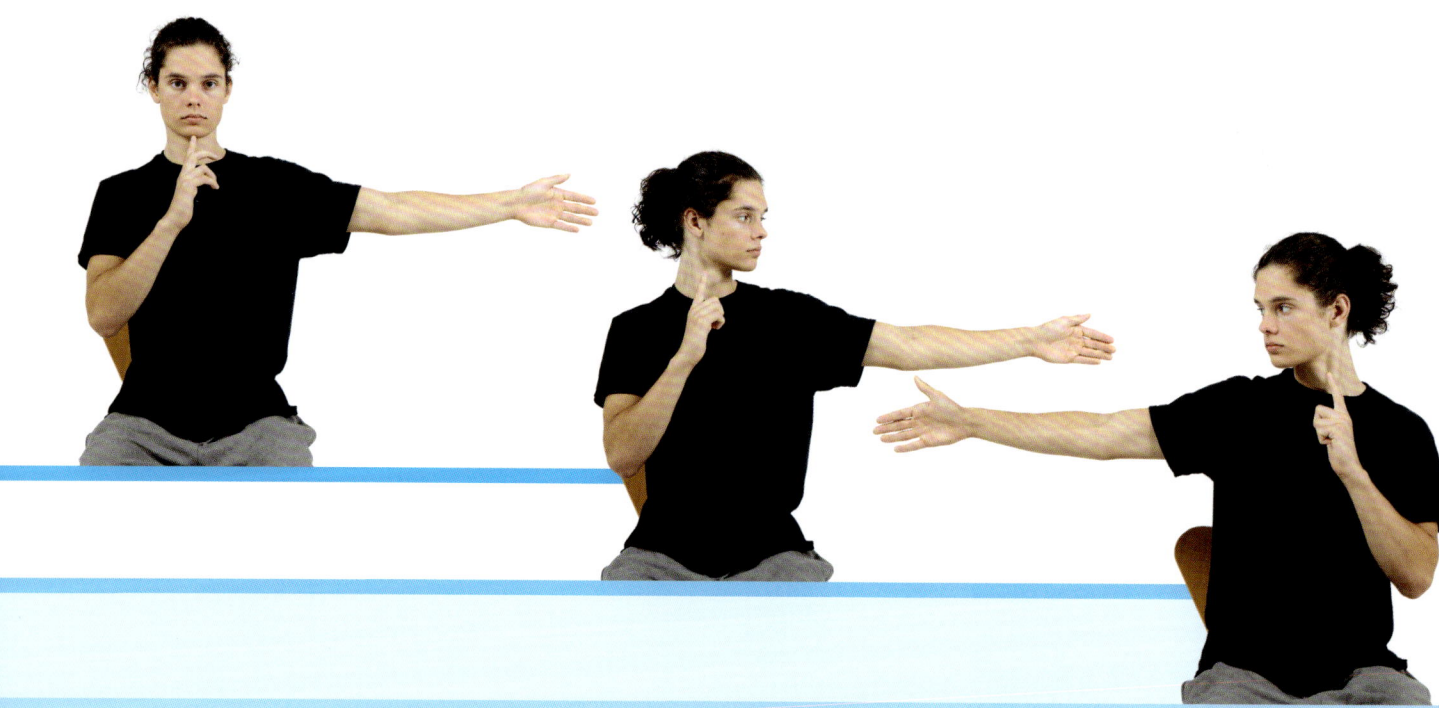

Table 5.2 Neck rotation results

You can easily turn beyond 45 degrees on either side	You can almost turn to 45 degrees on either side	You find it difficult to reach 45 degrees on either side
Your neck rotation is good. To help maintain this, try these exercises: **1.** Turn right, turn left (*see* p. 82) **2.** Back of neck stretch A or B (*see* p. 85 or p. 86) **3.** Lying down neck massage (*see* p. 92) Or try the Neck Option 1 or Option 2 sequences in table 9.3 on p. 120.	Your neck rotation is reasonable but can be improved. Try these exercises: **1.** Slide the chin in (*see* p. 83) **2.** Decompress your neck (*see* p. 88) **3.** Nodding neck massage (*see* p. 90) Or try the Neck Option 1 or Option 2 sequences in table 9.3 on p. 120 or the Office Worker Option 1 or Option 2 sequences in table 9.8 on p. 130.	You will feel better if you improve your neck mobility, so let's get started. Try these exercises: **1.** Upper back rotation seated or standing (*see* pp. 61–2) **2.** Release your neck (*see* p. 89) **3.** Rotating neck massage (*see* p. 91) Or try the Neck Option 1 or Option 2 sequences in table 9.3 on p. 120 or the Office Worker Option 1 or Option 2 sequences in table 9.8 on p. 130.

NECK SIDE-BENDING TEST

This simple test follows on from the one previously to give you an indication of your neck's current range of motion. It is easiest to assess how far you can side-bend your neck if you do the tests in front of a mirror:

1. Sit upright at the back of a stable chair.
2. Relax your shoulders down and keep your tummy in.
3. Breathe in and as you breathe out, slowly lower your head to one side. Gently lengthen your neck as you take your ear towards your shoulder. Don't turn your head and keep looking forward.
4. Stop the movement if you feel a pinching in your neck. The limitation of movement should come from muscle tightness on the opening side of the neck.
5. Ideally you should be able to side-bend your neck so your head is about a third to halfway (30 to 45 degrees) over to the side.
6. Repeat on the other side. Note down your results and refer to table 5.3 to assess your results.

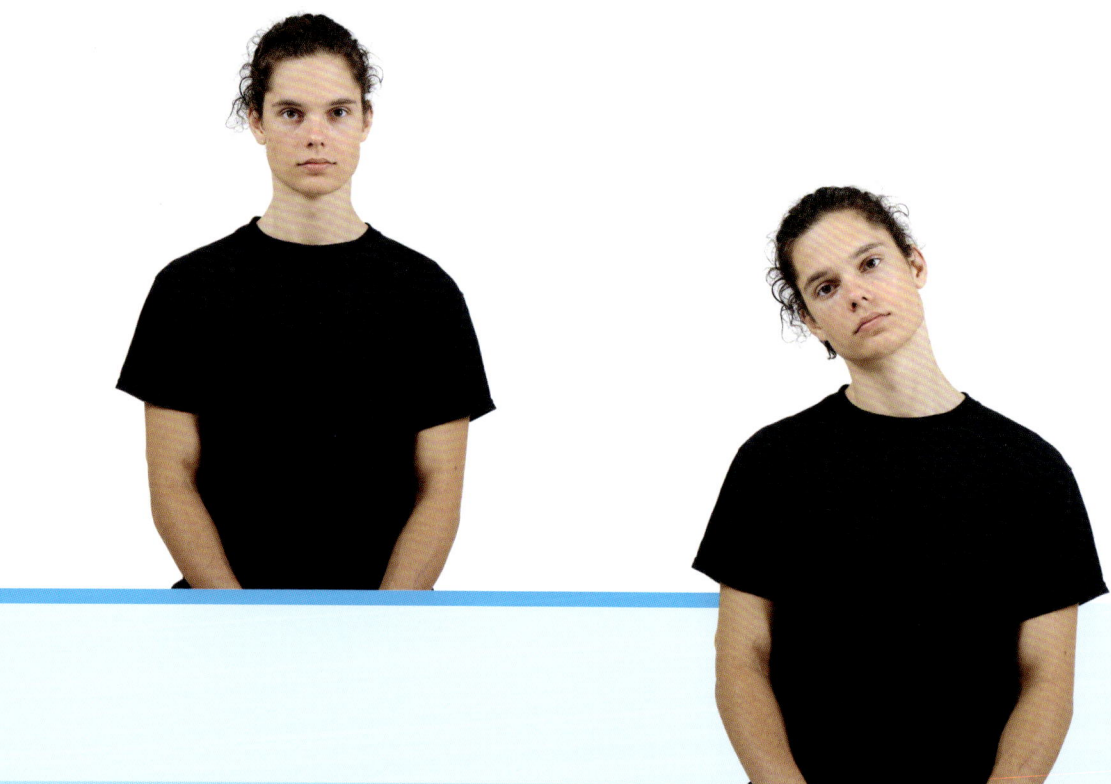

Table 5.3 Neck side-bending test results

You can almost bend to 45 degrees on either side	You can bend to 30 degrees on either side	You can only bend a little on both sides
Your neck side-bending is excellent. To help maintain this, try these exercises: **1.** Rib opener stretch (*see* p. 70) **2.** Pendulum swing behind (*see* p. 99) **3.** Release your neck (*see* p. 89) Or try the Neck Option 1 or Option 2 sequences in table 9.3 on p. 120.	Your neck side-bending is good but can be improved. Try these exercises: **1.** Upper back easer A or B (*see* p. 60 and p. 68) **2.** De-stress your neck (*see* p. 87) **3.** Nodding neck massage (*see* p. 90) Or try the Neck Option 1 or Option 2 sequences in table 9.3 on p. 120 or the Forward head and neck posture Option 1 or Option 2 sequences in table 9.24 on p. 162.	You will feel better if you improve your neck mobility, so let's get started. Try these exercises: **1.** De-stress your neck (*see* p. 87) **2.** Neck settling movements × 3 (*see* p. 81) **3.** Neck saucer glide (*see* p. 84) Or try the Neck Option 1 or Option 2 sequences in table 9.3 on p. 120 or the Forward head and neck posture Option 1 or Option 2 sequences in table 9.24 on p. 162.

SHOULDER BLADE REACH TESTS

The shoulders have a wide variety of movements, but the following three tests will give you a good idea of how tight your shoulders are and an indication of the most useful exercises to do to improve your shoulder function. Do all three tests on one side and then switch to the other side:

1. Stand or sit in a relaxed upright position with space behind your back.
2. Test 1: Up-the-back shoulder blade reach test – Keeping your shoulders relaxed, reach one arm up behind your back and try to touch the middle of the opposite shoulder blade. Aim for the area shown by the orange dot in figure 5.4a.
3. Test 2: Behind-the-head shoulder blade reach test – Relax your arm and then reach that arm behind your head and try and touch the middle of the opposite shoulder blade. Aim for the area shown by the orange dot in figure 5.4b.
4. Test 3: Across-and-behind shoulder blade reach test – Relax your arm again and then reach that arm across your chest and over and behind the opposite shoulder to try and touch the middle of the opposite shoulder blade. Aim for the area shown by the orange dot in figure 5.4c.
5. Now repeat all three tests with the other arm to assess the tightness of the opposite shoulder. Note down your results and refer to tables 5.4, 5.5 and 5.6 to assess your results.

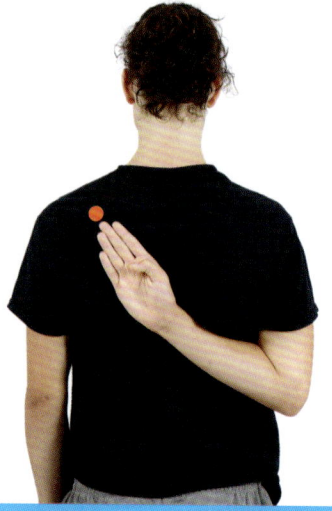

Figure 5.4a

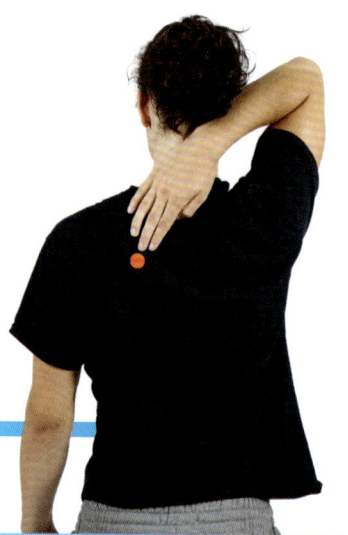

Figure 5.4b

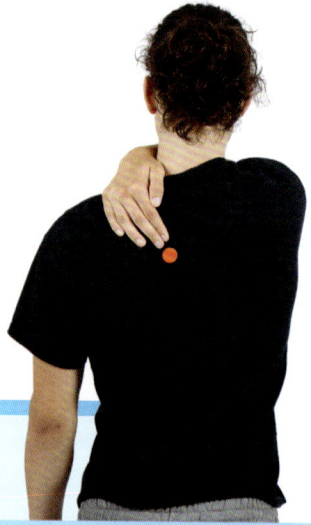

Figure 5.4c

Table 5.4 Up-the-back shoulder blade reach test results

You can easily reach the back of your shoulder blade	You can just reach the bottom of the opposite shoulder blade	You find it difficult to reach beyond your lower back
Your range of movement is excellent. To help maintain this, try these exercises: 1. Two-arm swipe (see p. 67) 2. One-arm forward hang, standing or seated (see p. 104) 3. Horizontal arm circles (see p. 96) Or try the Shoulder Option 1 or Option 2 sequences in table 9.4 on p. 122.	Your range of movement is reasonable but can be improved. Try these exercises: 1. Backward hang (see p. 107) 2. Pendulum swing behind (see p. 99) 3. Top of shoulder massage (see p. 112) Or try the Shoulder Option 1 or Option 2 sequences in table 9.4 on p. 122 or the Arthritic Shoulders Option 1 or Option 2 sequences in table 9.26 on p. 166.	You will feel better if you improve your shoulder mobility, so let's get started. Try these exercises: 1. Back scratcher (see p. 108) 2. Upper back easer A (see p. 60) 3. Shoulder cross-fibre massage (see p. 110) Or try the Shoulder Option 1 or Option 2 sequences in table 9.4 on p. 122 or the Arthritic Shoulders Option 1 or Option 2 sequences in table 9.26 on p. 166.

Table 5.5 Behind-the-head shoulder blade reach test results

You can easily reach the back of the opposite shoulder blade	You can just reach the top of the opposite shoulder blade	You find it difficult to reach beyond the back of your neck
Your range of movement is excellent. To help maintain this, try these exercises: 1. Pendulum swing front (*see* p. 98) 2. Shoulder blade squeezer (*see* p. 103) 3. Upper back massage (*see* p. 75) Or try the Shoulder Option 1 or Option 2 sequences in table 9.4 on p. 122.	Your range of movement is reasonable but can be improved. Try these exercises: 1. Upper back round and lift (*see* p. 66) 2. Two-arm forward hang, seated (*see* p. 71) 3. Shoulder rolling massage (*see* p. 109) Or try the Shoulder Option 1 or Option 2 sequences in table 9.4 on p. 122 or the Arthritic Shoulders Option 1 or Option 2 sequences in table 9.26 on p. 166.	You will feel better if you improve your shoulder mobility, so let's get started. Try these exercises: 1. Across-body hang, standing or seated (*see* p. 105) 2. Chest lift (*see* p. 65) 3. Shoulder blade muscle massage (*see* p. 111) Or try the Shoulder Option 1 or Option 2 sequences in table 9.4 on p. 122 or the Arthritic Shoulders Option 1 or Option 2 sequences in table 9.26 on p. 166.

Table 5.6 Across-and-behind shoulder blade reach test results

You can easily reach the middle of the opposite shoulder blade	You can just reach the top of the back of the opposite shoulder blade	You find it difficult to reach the top of the opposite shoulder blade
Your range of movement is excellent. To help maintain this, try these exercises: 1. Upper back rotation, seated (see p. 62) 2. Push forward, pull back (see p. 97) 3. Spinal muscle massage (see p. 74) Or try the Shoulder Option 1 or Option 2 sequences in table 9.4 on p. 122.	Your range of movement is reasonable but can be improved. Try these exercises: 1. Rib opener stretch (see p. 70) 2. One-arm forward hang, standing or seated (see p. 104) 3. Shoulder cross-fibre massage (see p. 110) Or try the Shoulder Option 1 or Option 2 sequences in table 9.4 on p. 122 or the Arthritic Shoulders Option 1 or Option 2 sequences in table 9.26 on p. 166.	You will feel better if you improve your shoulder mobility, so let's get started. Try these exercises: 1. Rib release (see p. 64) 2. Cross-body reach (see p. 100) 3. Side of back massage (see p. 76) Or try the Shoulder Option 1 or Option 2 sequences in table 9.4 on p. 122 or the Arthritic Shoulders Option 1 or Option 2 sequences in table 9.26 on p. 166.

PART 2

EXERCISES AND SEQUENCES

All the movements and stretches in this book can be done while standing or sitting. A sturdy, stable chair without arms will give you the greatest freedom for movement. If a chair has arms you can still do the seated movements but some of the exercises may be slightly restricted. You could also use the edge of a sofa or bed as long as they are reasonably firm. When sitting down, your hips should be at the same level or slightly higher than your knees.

You don't need any special equipment for the movements, stretches and self-massages, as a pole and a massage roller you have at home can be used. If you do not have a massage roller, you could also improvise using a bottle of frozen water, a tennis ball in a sock or a rolling pin with a hand towel wrapped and secured around it. (*see* p. 10 for more on equipment). Only one exercise and one massage is shown lying down (*see* p. 63 and p. 92), so you don't need to buy an exercise mat; you can certainly use a mat if you have one anyway, but if not, you can use your bed, provided that your mattress is firm and doesn't dip.

When doing the movements, stretches or self-massages, the maximum space needed in your room or along a wall is a few centimetres longer than the length of your arms when they are fully extended. Many exercises and massages, for example, neck stretches, can be done with no extra space.

Chapters 6, 7 and 8 focus on movements, stretches and self-massages for the upper back, neck and shoulders. You can either just experiment and try out some exercises, and find what works for you and what you like doing or visit the tightness tests in Chapter 5 for a starting point and exercise recommendations. This is especially helpful if you have areas you know are particularly tight or painful.

The movements, stretches and massages are particularly powerful when they're combined, so in Chapter 9 you will find some suggested sequences for specific scenarios or areas of concern. In fact, you can choose to combine any number of elements, but make sure you always include an upper back exercise or stretch (*see* Chapter 6), because mobility in this part of your body is essential for comfort and balanced function. It is also sensible to do settling movements (*see* pp. 59, 60, 81, 96 and 97) after each stretch/hang to help the muscles to relax into their new length. This helps to soothe them and to reduce the likelihood of cramp.

So, whether you're a gamer with tech neck or a golfer with a sore shoulder, you're sure to find relief if you follow the advice and Make Movement Your Medicine.

6 UPPER BACK MOVEMENTS, STRETCHES AND SELF-MASSAGES

UPPER BACK MOVEMENTS, STRETCHES AND SELF-MASSAGES

Your upper back probably suffers from sedentary modern living, particularly if you sit at a desk all day or are constantly looking at a screen. Fortunately, the exercises in this section are simple and effective, and will help relieve any pain you have and keep your upper back functioning well.

Remember:
- You don't need to do all the movements, stretches and self-massages in this section at once, and you don't have to do them in any particular order.
- Identify the exercises you find most effective and enjoyable, or use the tightness tests (*see* pp. 42–53) to identify which you need most, and build them into your daily routine.
- It is good to always start with the three essential upper back exercises (*see* p 116) as these are vital for upper back comfort and function, but will also take strain off your neck and shoulders.
- It is a good idea to do the upper back settling movements after each stretch. (see pp. 59 and 60) to settle the joints and muscles.
- All the movements, stretches and self-massages in this section are designed to keep your upper back mobile or, if you have pain in your upper back, to make it more comfortable.
- When doing any of these exercises, try to keep your tummy pulled in and – most importantly – don't forget to breathe.
- It is fine to work towards pain, but don't work through it. Even if you can only work in a very small, pain-free range, it's still worth doing.
- If your muscles do feel sore or ache from the exercises, it may be helpful to apply heat or a cold pack and to gently massage them, as this will help them adjust to healthy movement.

EXERCISE SYMBOLS

To help you identify whether an exercise needs any equipment, we have included a **P** symbol for stretches that require a pole, and an **R** symbol for self-massages that require a roller.

Table 6.1 Upper back exercises quick reference

Page number	Movements	Benefits
59	Rib shifter (settling movement)	Releases stiffness and aching in the upper back and ribs
60	Upper back easer A (settling movement)	Ensures well-aligned sitting posture and can help to reduce dowager's hump
61	Upper back rotation, standing	Reduces stiffness in the upper back and helps neck and shoulder comfort
62	Upper back rotation, seated	Reduces stiffness in the upper back and helps neck and shoulder comfort
63	Upper back rotation, lying	Reduces stiffness in the upper back and helps neck and shoulder comfort
64	Rib release	Releases stiffness and aching around your ribs and spine
65	Chest lift	Gets the area between your shoulder blades moving gently
66	Upper back round and lift	Restores movement and eases stiffness in your ribcage and upper back
67	Two-arm swipe	Reduces stiffness in your ribcage and spine, and softens tightness in your neck and shoulders
68	Upper back easer B	Helps to correct or prevent a rounded upper back and mobilises the spine between your shoulder blades
Stretches		
69	Desk chest stretch	Releases tight chest muscles, helping the shoulders not to round
70	Rib opener stretch	Relieves stiffness in the side of your ribcage and upper back
71	Two-arm forward hang, seated	Helps you to have a more comfortable, balanced and well-aligned sitting posture
72	Chest and shoulder release A	Helps to open the shoulders, reducing rounding by releasing shortened and tightened chest muscles
73	Chest and shoulder release B	Helps to open the shoulders, reducing rounding by releasing shortened and tightened chest muscles
Self-massages		
74	Spinal muscle massage	Releases tight muscles either side of the spine
75	Upper back massage	Unsticks tight muscles between your shoulder blades and spine
76	Side of back massage	Helps to release back muscles, improving back and shoulder mobility

UPPER BACK MOVEMENTS, STRETCHES AND SELF-MASSAGES

MOVEMENTS

Rib shifter

This settling movement is useful for releasing stiffness and aching in the upper back and ribs. It is one of the upper back settling movements that should be done after upper back stretches to soothe and calm the muscles and joints into their new positions.

- Sit in neutral posture (*see* p. 38) on a reasonably firm chair with your hands on the sides of your ribs, and your shoulders and arms relaxed.
- Gently push your ribs out to the right side, and then to the left side, easing to comfortable end points.
- Keep your weight even through your buttocks, and your hips level and still, to avoid rocking. Your head and neck should be gently drawn back with your ears over your shoulders.
- Repeat 2–5 times on both sides.
- **Remember that wherever your body is most tight is where you will feel it first.**

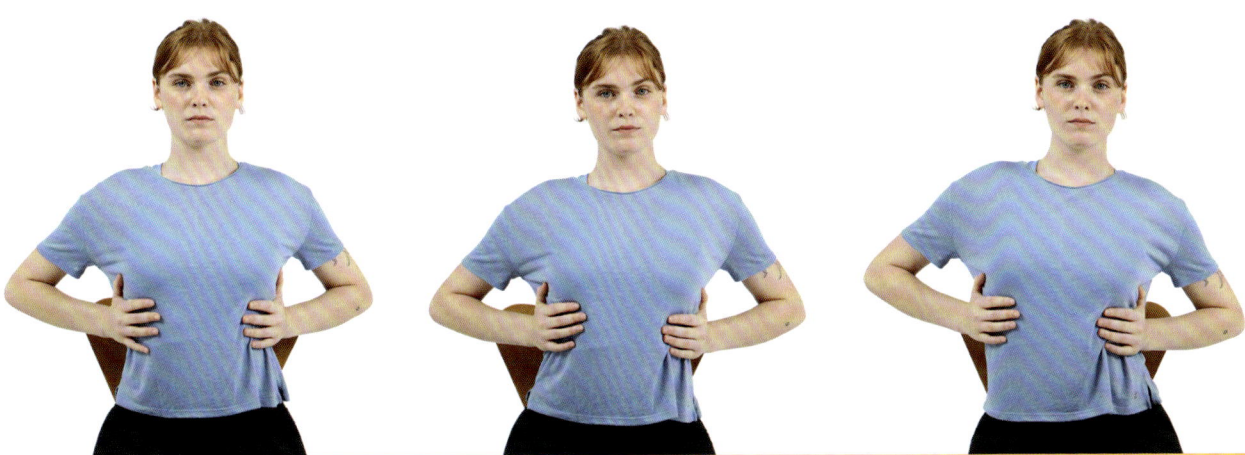

You should feel a gentle movement and stretching sensation in your ribs, and your tummy muscles working to support the movement. Some tightness is quite normal and by doing the movement regularly, the tightness will reduce.

Upper back easer A

As well as helping you find a comfortable, balanced and well-aligned sitting posture, this settling movement helps to reduce or prevent a 'dowager's hump' (a lump at the base of the neck) or the creases in the back of your neck, which come from slouching.

- Sit in neutral posture (*see* p. 38) on a reasonably firm chair with some space behind your back. Rest your hands on your thighs.
- Gently curve your whole spine towards the back of the chair by pulling your tummy in.
- Come back to the start position, then lift the middle of your chest bone towards the ceiling, creating a slight hollow in your back between your shoulder blades.
- This is a gentle flowing movement but keep your shoulders down and try not to let your head come too far forwards.
- Repeat 2–5 times.
- **To keep your ribs down, sigh deeply. This relaxes your lower ribs and stops them sticking out.**

You should feel this in your upper back, particularly in the muscles either side of your spine, but you are also likely to feel it in your chest muscles, the front part of your shoulders and maybe in your upper tummy muscles too.

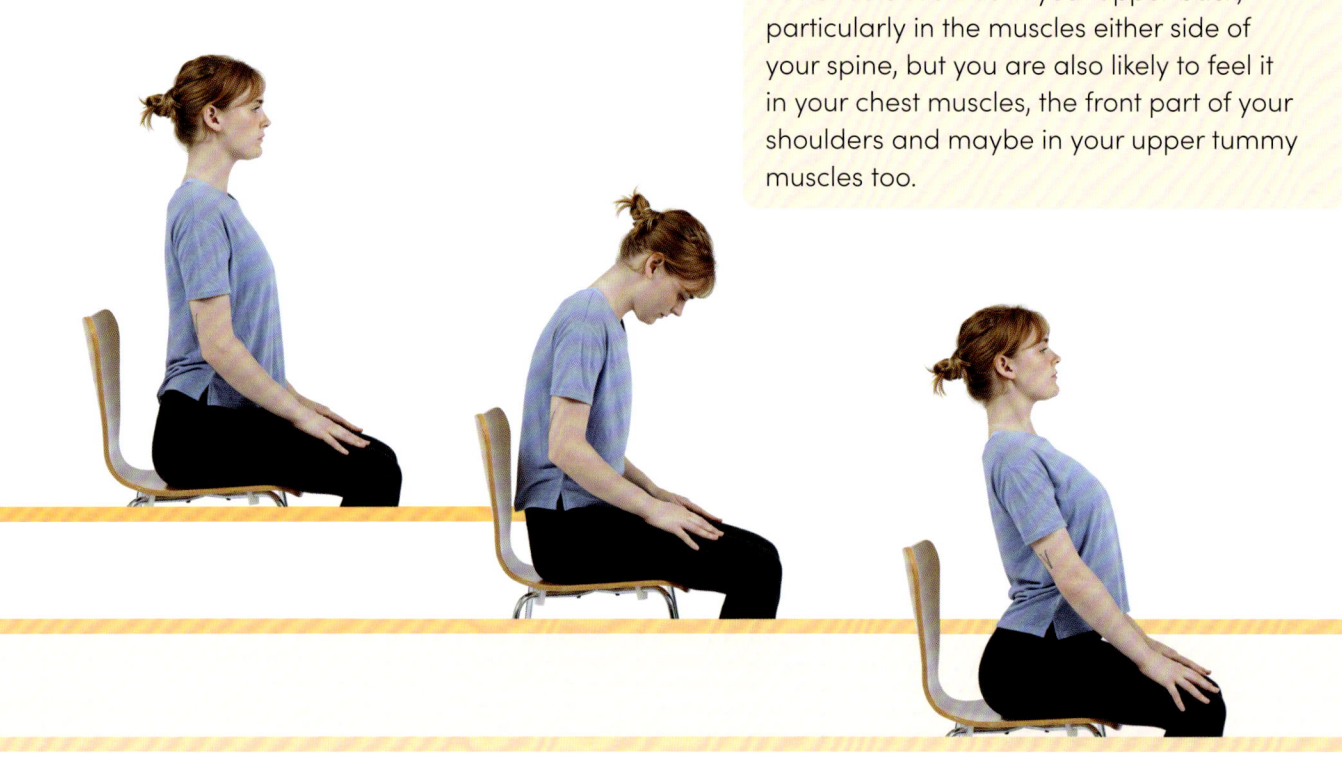

UPPER BACK MOVEMENTS, STRETCHES AND SELF-MASSAGES

Upper back rotation, standing

This exercise can be done almost anywhere – while walking the dog, waiting in a queue or taking a break on a long car or plane journey. It reduces stiffness in the upper back and helps to take the strain off your neck and shoulders.

- Stand upright in a neutral posture (*see* p. 35) with your hips facing forwards and your right leg slightly out in front of you.
- Place your right-hand thumb on the middle of your chest bone and your fingers on your chin.
- Breathe in and then, as you breathe out, turn your upper body to the right, going as far as is comfortable without forcing the movement. Think of the middle of your chest leading the turn, and your chin and head going with it.
- Keep your hips still and facing forwards, and your neck and shoulders relaxed.
- At the end of your turn, take a big breath in and, as you breathe out, try to turn a little further, but still without forcing the movement.
- At your new end point, take another breath in and then return to the start position as you breathe out.
- Repeat 2–3 times to the right side, then swap your legs round and do the same to the left side.
- **Keep your hips and legs still. Stay tall and draw your head back so that your ears are over your shoulders.**

You should feel a gentle twisting and turning sensation in your spine and ribcage. There shouldn't be any straining in your lower back or neck, but you should notice your tummy muscles working to help stabilise your lower back. After several repetitions you should feel a release of tension, and easier breathing and movement.

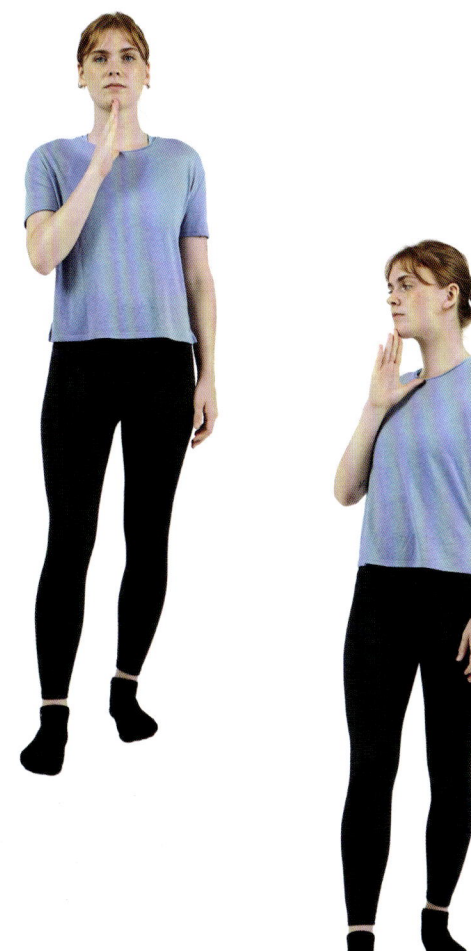

MAKE MOVEMENT YOUR MEDICINE

Upper back rotation, seated

This is a perfect exercise to do anytime you are seated, for example at your desk or when on a plane. It reduces stiffness in the ribcage and spine, which in turn helps take stress off the neck and shoulders.

- Sit tall in neutral posture (*see* p. 38) with your right hand on your chest and your fingertips touching your chin. It can be helpful to place a ball or cushion between your legs.
- Lengthen through your spine as you gently turn your upper body to the right, keeping your hand on your chest. The middle of your chest leads the movement and your nose and chin turn in line with it.
- Keep your chin level, your hips and buttocks level and still, and your lower ribs down.
- At the end of your turn, take a big breath in and, as you breathe out, try to turn a little further, but still without forcing the movement.
- At your new end point, take another breath in and then return to the start position as you breathe out.
- Repeat 2–5 times on each side.
- **Keep your shoulders down, your ears above your shoulders and your chin level. Your legs, hips and lower back should all be still.**

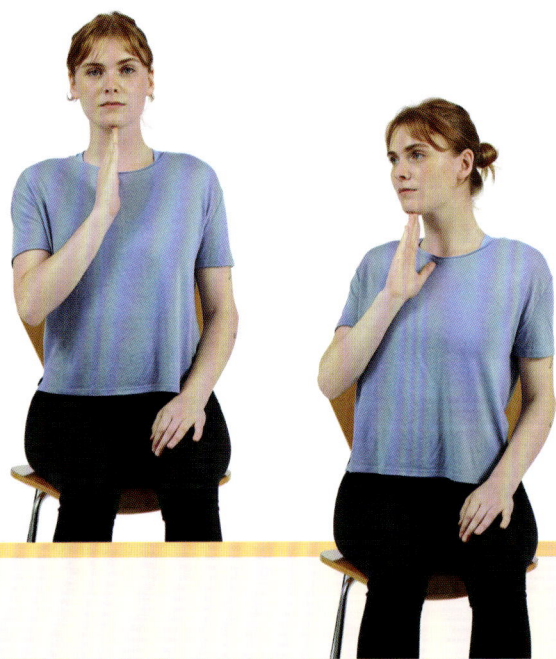

You should feel a gentle twisting and turning sensation in your spine, chest and ribcage. There shouldn't be any straining in your lower back or neck, but you should notice your tummy muscles working to help stabilise your lower back. After several repetitions you should feel a release of tension, and easier breathing and movement.

Upper back rotation, lying

The advantage of this exercise is that it doesn't place any weight on the spine – you can even do it lying in bed. It reduces stiffness in the ribs and spine and also helps take strain off the neck and shoulders.

- Lie on your left side, with your head in line with your spine on a pillow at a comfortable height and your shoulders, hips and knees stacked in a straight line slightly out in front of you, at a 45-degree angle to your body.
- Keep your spine lengthened and your top hip still and lengthened away from your ribs. Your head should be facing forward.
- With both of your legs closed together in front of you at 90 degrees at the knee.
- Place your left hand on your right thigh. Place your right hand on your lower ribs.
- Gently pull your tummy in and take a deep breath in through your nose.
- As you start to breathe out as if blowing a kiss, rotate through your spine to turn the front of your chest and head towards the ceiling.
- Only go as far as is comfortable, keeping your hips and legs still. Then take another deep breath in through the nose and as you breathe out gently rotate a little further.
- At your new end point, take another breath in and then return to the start position as you breathe out.
- Repeat the whole process 2–3 times on each side.
- **Keep your tummy in and your head and neck relaxed, as though you're sunbathing on your pillow. Your legs and hips should be still and you should keep tall through your spine. You should not feel this movement in your lower back. If you do, stop and reposition yourself.**

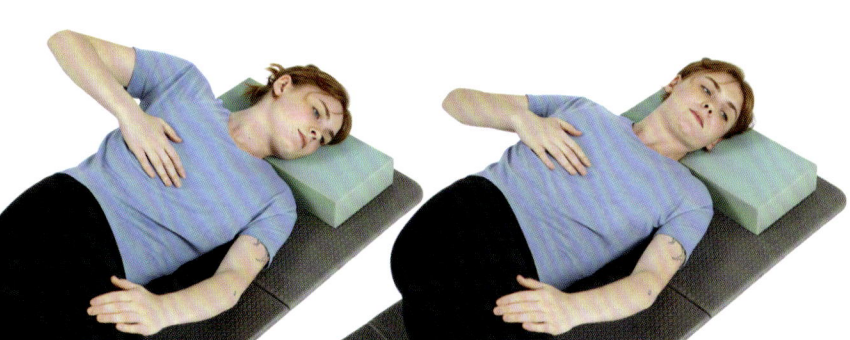

MORE ROTATIONS

You can also do the same exercise with your top hand in different positions. Try it with your hand on your upper chest or behind your head. This emphasises the movement and takes the stretch into different areas of your upper body.

You should feel stretching in your mid-back which you may experience as gentle pulling. This will gradually release as the area relaxes and you feel a gentle twisting sensation through your spine and ribcage. You will then feel able to naturally rotate a little further. You shouldn't feel any pinching strain in your lower back or neck. Try to feel the muscles in your tummy and buttocks engaging to stabilise your lower back. By repeating this exercise you can release tension in your back and make your breathing and movement easier.

Rib release

This exercise releases stiffness and aching around your ribs and spine. It is perfect for anyone sitting with their upper back held still for much of the day, such as desk workers, drivers and commuters.

- Sit in neutral posture (*see* p. 38) on a reasonably firm chair.
- Draw your head back so your ears are over your shoulders and keep your chin level. Fix your eyes on a point straight ahead of you.
- Hold your hands together in front of you, tucking your arms and elbows in close to your ribs.
- Keep your head still and face forwards as you slowly slide your elbows around your middle to the right-hand side. Ideally your front elbow should move round to be in line with your tummy button and your back elbow round towards your spine.
- Go as far as is comfortable and then repeat to the left-hand side, keeping your weight even on both buttocks and your tummy in. The movement should be smooth and continuous.
- Repeat 2–5 times.
- **With your ears above your shoulders, keep the back of your neck long, and your chest and head still but relaxed.**

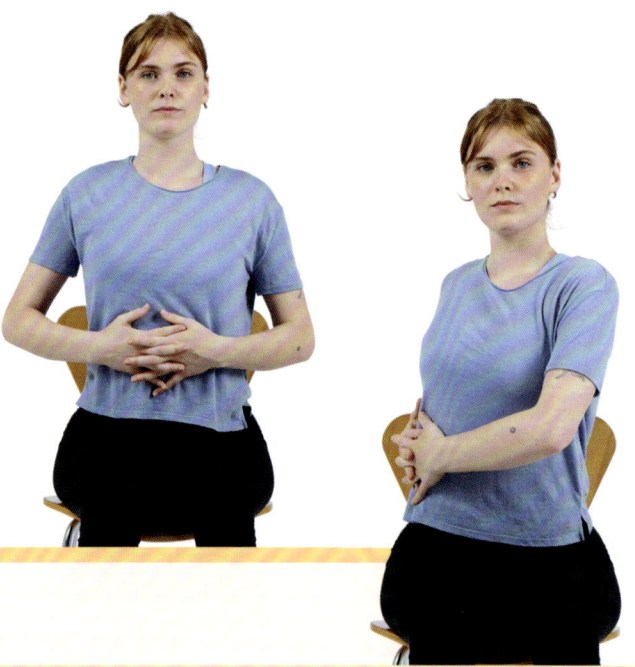

You should feel a gentle stretch around your ribcage and you may also feel your mid spine gently twisting. Your lower back should be still, and you will feel your tummy and buttocks muscles working to stabilise your lower body.

UPPER BACK MOVEMENTS, STRETCHES AND SELF-MASSAGES

Chest lift

To reduce stiffness, this exercise gets the area between your shoulder blades moving gently.

- Stand or sit in neutral posture (see p. 35 or p. 38) with some space behind your back, holding your hands together behind your back. Relax your shoulders.
- Lengthen both arms downwards, and at the same time lift and slide the middle of your chest up as you breathe out.
- Your shoulder blades will squeeze together and you will create a small hollow in your upper back.
- Return to the start position.
- Repeat 2–5 times.
- **The chest lift will be small. The key here is keeping your shoulders down and ribs relaxed.**

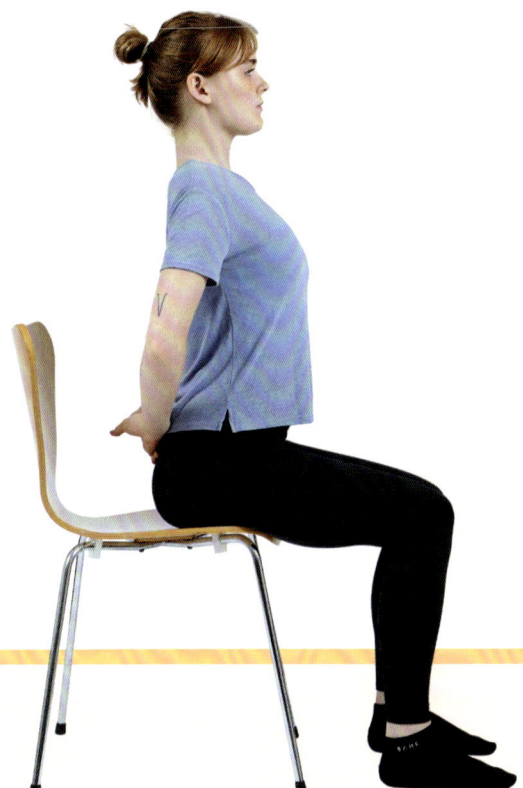

After doing this exercise you will feel lighter and freer, but while you're doing it you should observe a squeezing and tightening around your shoulder blades as they draw in and down. Your upper back muscles should contract and then relax again as they work to create the movement. You may feel a slight pulling sensation across the front of your shoulders, just below your ribs and in the front of your neck. Similarly, you may feel the muscles in your arms lengthening as you stretch them down your back.

MAKE MOVEMENT YOUR MEDICINE

ⓟ Upper back round and lift

Sedentary living and lack of regular climbing and reaching movements causes stiffness in the upper back. If you want to restore movement and ease stiffness in your ribcage and upper back, try this exercise.

- Sit tall in neutral posture (see p. 38) on a reasonably firm chair, with some space behind your back.
- Place a pole vertically in front of you, holding it with both hands at about chest height.
- Keeping your arms straight, gently curve your spine towards the back of the chair and lean the pole away from you.
- Bend your arms and bring the pole in towards you, lifting your chest as if you're sliding it up the pole. You are trying to get a slight arch in your back, between your shoulder blades.
- Repeat the movement 2–5 times, slowly flowing from one position to the other.
- **Relax your shoulders and don't let your lower ribs stick out. Try to keep your head drawn back and your chin level.**

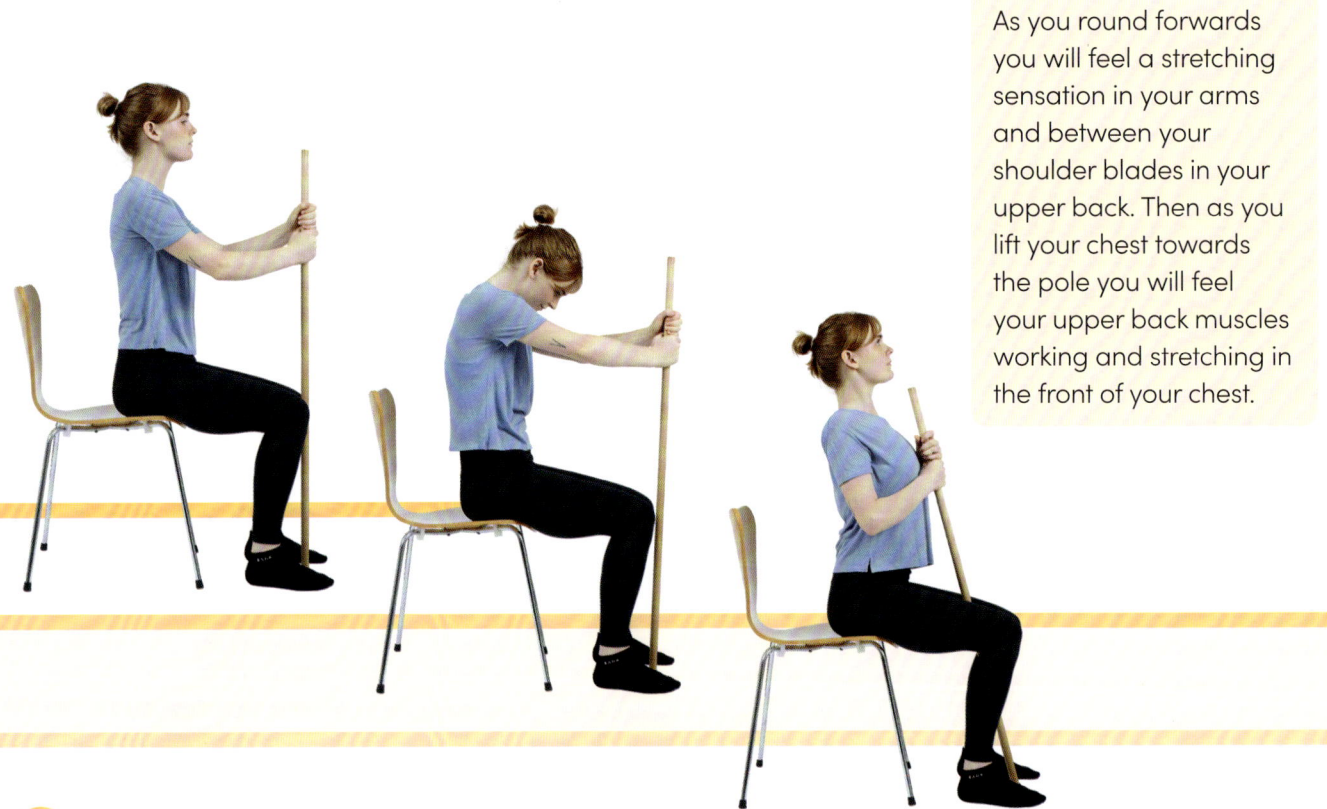

As you round forwards you will feel a stretching sensation in your arms and between your shoulder blades in your upper back. Then as you lift your chest towards the pole you will feel your upper back muscles working and stretching in the front of your chest.

UPPER BACK MOVEMENTS, STRETCHES AND SELF-MASSAGES

P Two-arm swipe

This is designed to reduce stiffness in your ribcage and spine, as well as softening tightness in your neck and shoulders. It is an exercise that is pleasantly reviving for anyone sitting for much of the day.

- Sit in neutral posture (*see* p. 38) on a reasonably firm chair.
- Place a pole vertically directly in front of you, holding it with both hands at chest height.
- Keeping your arms straight, let their weight be taken by your pole.
- Keep your eyes fixed on a point in front of you as you take your arms around to the right-hand side, as far as you can without straining.
- Smoothly move back through the starting position and to the left-hand side.
- Move continuously and repeat 2–5 times.
- **Keep your head and neck drawn gently back and your chin level. Try to keep your ribs relaxed down to stop them sticking out and be sure to keep your arms straight throughout the movement.**

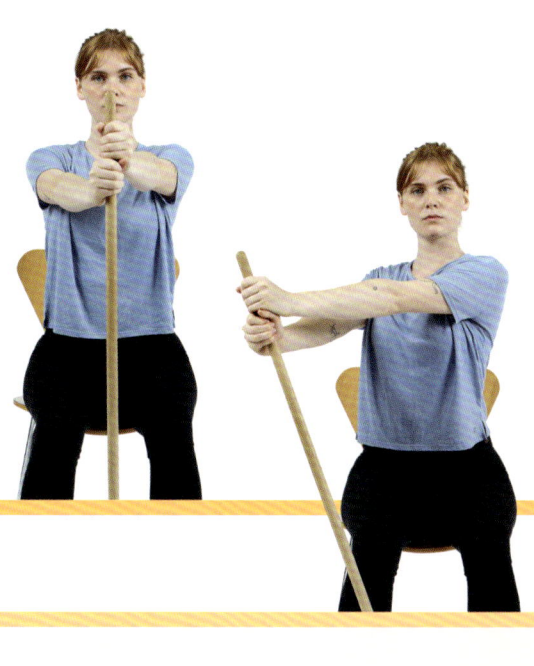
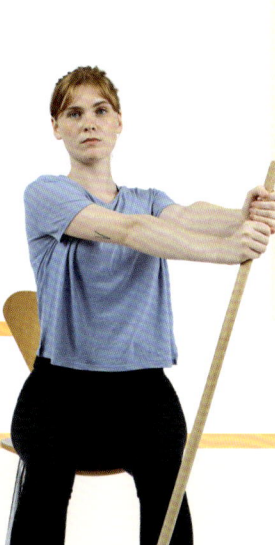

You will feel a smooth, swinging and twisting action in your back, ribs and waist. With each repetition the muscles around your ribs and spine should loosen. You may also feel a relieving stretch in your shoulders, arms and chest – like light tension melting away – and your tummy and buttock muscles squeezing or contracting as they work.

Upper back easer B

This exercise helps to correct or prevent a rounded upper back and to mobilise the spine between your shoulder blades. If you don't have a ball, you can use a similar prop, such as a cushion.

- Sit in neutral posture (*see* p. 38) on a reasonably firm chair.
- Place a soft ball or something similar between the lowest part of your shoulder blades and the back of your chair.
- Start by lifting your chest up and over the ball to gently curve your spine, keeping your tummy in, your hips and buttocks level and still, and your lower ribs down.
- Try to create a small hollow in your upper back. It is normal for this area to feel stiff and to only achieve a small movement.
- Return to an upright position and continue the movement by curving yourself forwards over an imaginary large beach ball on your lap. You will feel your spine round backwards as you curve your trunk forwards.
- Repeat 2–5 times, with the movement gently flowing.
- **Keep your feet evenly weighted, your buttocks and hips still, and if you need to stop your ribs from sticking out, give a big sigh. The movements should be smooth. Try to stop your chin lifting up or jamming down.**

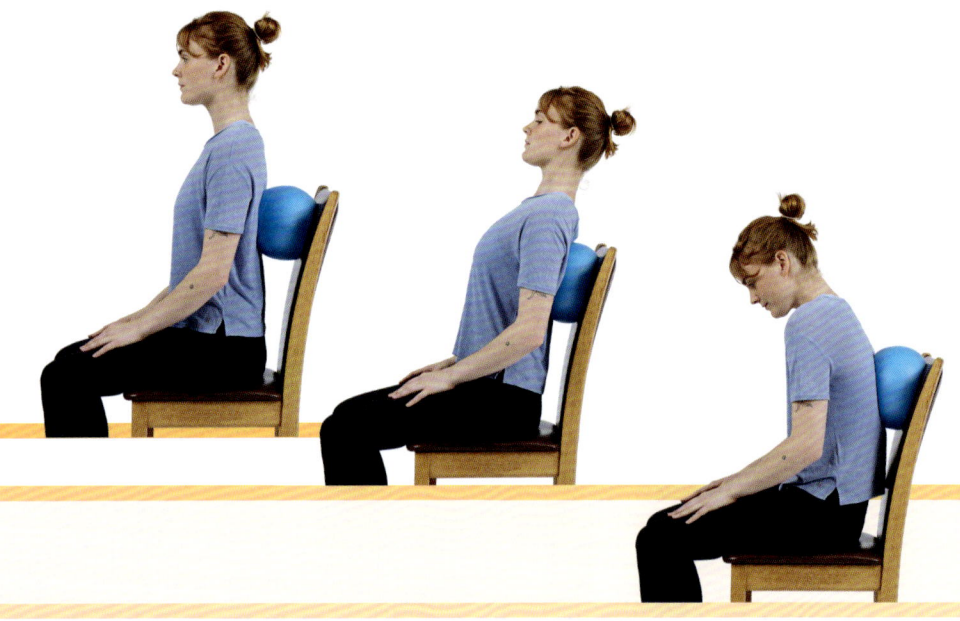

You will feel your spine arching gently backwards and your chest lifting as your upper body rounds over the ball. Then, as you come forwards, you will feel your spine rounding and your chest lowering – but don't go too low. It might feel as if your back is having a massage as the tightness eases with the flowing movement. You should feel the ball or cushion behind you pushing into your back.

STRETCHES

Desk chest stretch

Stretching is one of the best things you can do to keep your upper body functioning optimally. This exercise releases tight chest muscles caused by prolonged use of laptops, phones or tablets, or studying or driving.

- Sit in neutral posture (*see* p. 38) on a reasonably firm chair facing or side on to a table or desk. Plant your feet on the ground hip-width apart.
- Rest the palm of your right hand against the front edge of the table and your left hand on your thigh. Keep your head and neck gently drawn back and your tummy in.
- Slowly lengthen your right arm by sliding your hand along the edge of the table.
- As your arm straightens, turn your palm towards the ceiling and apply a little pressure against the edge of the table.
- At the same time gently turn the middle of your chest bone to the left-hand side to create an opening chest stretch on the lengthened right-arm side and hold for up to 30 seconds.
- Repeat 2–5 times on each side.
- **Keep your ears over your shoulders, your ribs relaxed, your hips and buttocks still and your chin level.**

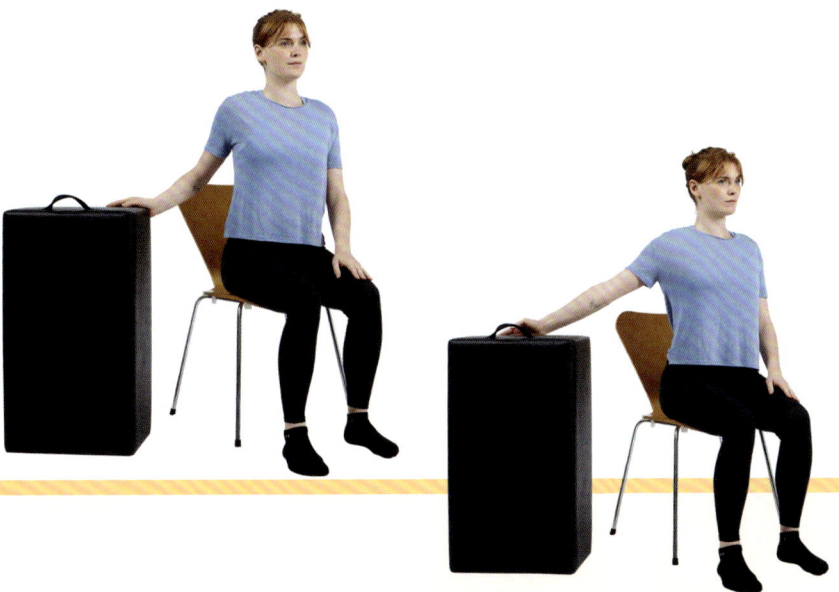

You will feel a gradual pulling as you straighten your arm and turn your chest. As you hold the stretch in the muscles in your chest, shoulder arm and forearm, the tightness will gradually release.

🅟 Rib opener stretch

This exercise is designed to help to relieve stiffness in the side of your ribcage and to mobilise your spine. Getting your ribcage to move more freely also helps you to breathe more easily. This is particularly helpful for people who have to sit or stand for much of the day or for people with a cough or asthma.

- Sit in neutral posture (*see* p. 38) on a reasonably firm chair with your feet hip width apart.
- Place a pole vertically at arms' length out to the right in line with your hips, with one end on the floor, holding it in your left hand at shoulder level. (The pole can be placed on a raised surface as shown if it is too short.) Then lean it across the front of your body.
- With your left hand, hold the pole as far up as is comfortable. Your palm should face forwards and your thumb downwards. Try to keep your ears over your shoulders and keep looking forwards with your tummy in.
- Gently extend your left arm up and over your head, still holding the pole, as far as is comfortable as you lift and curve your ribcage out to the left-hand side.
- Hold for up to 30 seconds while breathing.
- To return to the start position, keep your tummy in and gently pull your ribs down on the left-hand side, towards your hip, using your waist muscles.
- Repeat 2–3 times on each side.
- **Try to avoid squashing your ribs. Keep your head and chest facing forwards and your weight even through your buttocks to avoid rocking.**

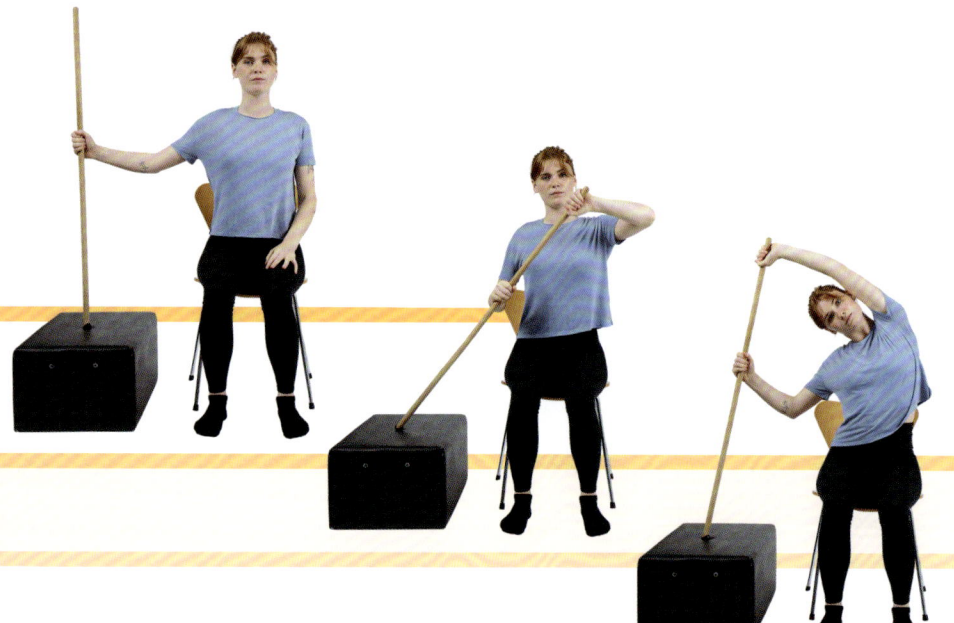

As you reach further over with the pole, you will feel a gradual increase in the stretch. This will feel like pulling or lengthening in the muscles through the extended side of your body. At the end of the stretch you will feel lighter and freer in your upper body

Ⓟ Two-arm forward hang, seated

This exercise will help you to have a more comfortable, balanced and well-aligned sitting posture, especially if your chest and shoulder muscles are causing you to slump forwards. This is beneficial for anyone whose posture suffers from using modern tech or anyone who is in one position for long periods of the day.

- Sit in neutral posture (*see* p. 38) on a reasonably firm chair.
- Place a pole vertically directly in front of you, holding the pole with both hands as high as you comfortably can. (The pole can be placed on a raised surface as shown if it is too short.).
- Keeping your arms straight and your chest lifted, lean forwards until you feel a gentle hanging stretch around and under your shoulders. It will also stretch into your upper back.
- Let your pole take the weight of your arms as you lean forwards to a level that is comfortable, keeping your ears over your shoulders and your chin slightly tucked.
- To increase the hanging stretch, activate your muscles by softly drawing your shoulder blades down or pushing the pole into the floor.
- Hold for up to 30 seconds with your arms straight, but not overextended at your elbows.
- Repeat 2–3 times.
- **Keep your head and neck drawn back, your ears over your shoulders, your chin slightly tucked and your ribs relaxed so they don't stick out. This is a gentle hanging stretch, so be careful not to overdo it.**

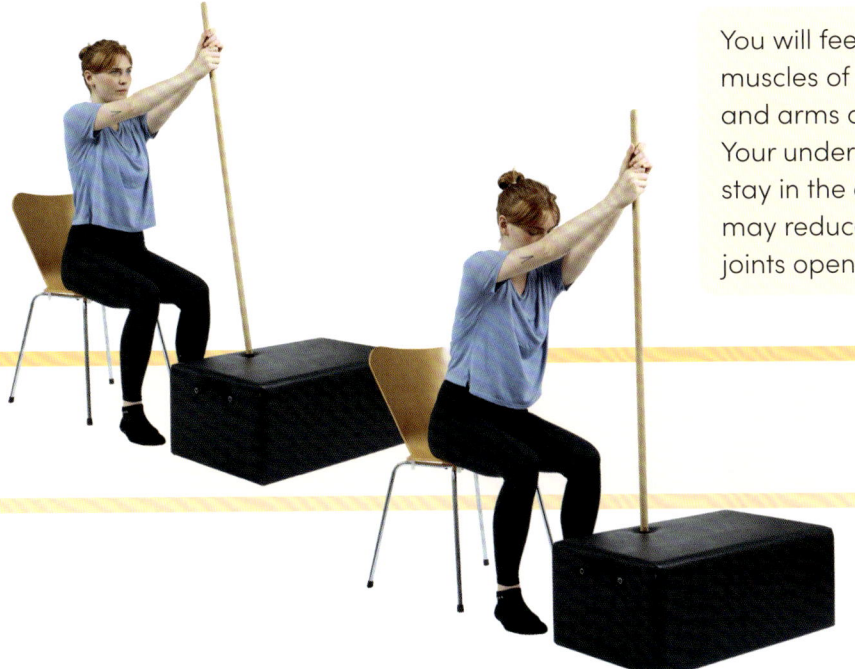

You will feel a pulling sensation in the muscles of your upper back, shoulders and arms as they lengthen and stretch. Your underarms will gently open. As you stay in the end position, these feelings may reduce or fade as the muscles and joints open and release.

MAKE MOVEMENT YOUR MEDICINE

🅟 Chest and shoulder release A

This stretch is designed to release the shortened and tightened chest muscles that can cause forward and rounded shoulders and a hunched back.

Note: This stretch is not suitable if you struggle to get into the start position or if it causes joint pain. If that is the case for you, go to chest and shoulder release B (see p. 73).

- Sit in neutral posture (*see* p. 38) on a reasonably firm chair.
- Hold a pole across your shoulders behind your upper back, not on your neck. Lengthen your arms along the pole with your palms facing forwards.
- Keep your head and neck drawn back and your tummy gently pulled in.
- Keep gently pressing your hands forwards into the pole and slowly turn your chest a small amount to the right and then the left repeating these small movements for up to 30 seconds.
- To increase the stretch, let your elbows bend a little so that your hands come a little closer together.
- **Keep your shoulders and ribs down to avoid arching your back, lengthen through your spine, and keep your hips, buttocks and head still.**

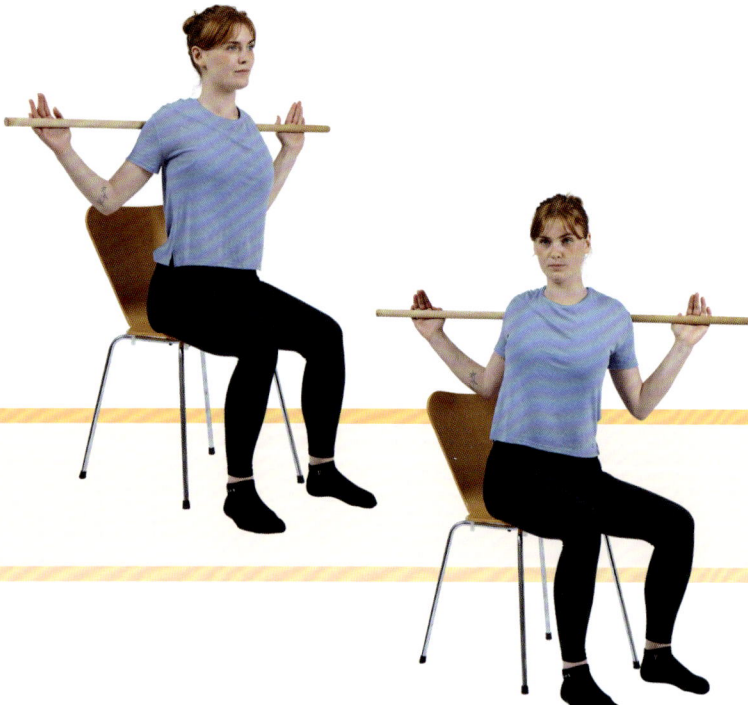

You will feel a dull, pulling feeling throughout your chest, and in your arms and shoulders, but as you continue with the stretch, try to relax into it to gain a feeling of your chest and shoulder muscles opening. It will make you more free and able to achieve good posture.

UPPER BACK MOVEMENTS, STRETCHES AND SELF-MASSAGES

P Chest and shoulder release B

If you find it difficult to have both arms opened along the pole and the pole behind your back as in the previous exercise, then this is a simpler alternative.

- Stand tall in a neutral posture (see p. 35) with your feet shoulder-width apart and your right foot slightly further forwards than your left.
- Place a pole vertically to your right, in line with your hip. (The pole can be placed on a raised surface as shown if it is too short.).
- Hold it with your right hand as high up as you comfortably can. Your arm should be straight, but not over-extended at your elbow.
- Keeping the base of the pole on the floor, slowly and smoothly move your arm backwards until most of the pole is behind you, and you feel a stretch in the front of your chest and shoulder. Keep looking forwards with your hips square and still.
- Hold at the end point for up to 30 seconds, before coming back to the start position.
- Repeat up to 4 times on each side.
- **Keep your head and neck gently drawn back, your chin level, your upper body and shoulders relaxed, and your ribs relaxed, too, to avoid them sticking out.**

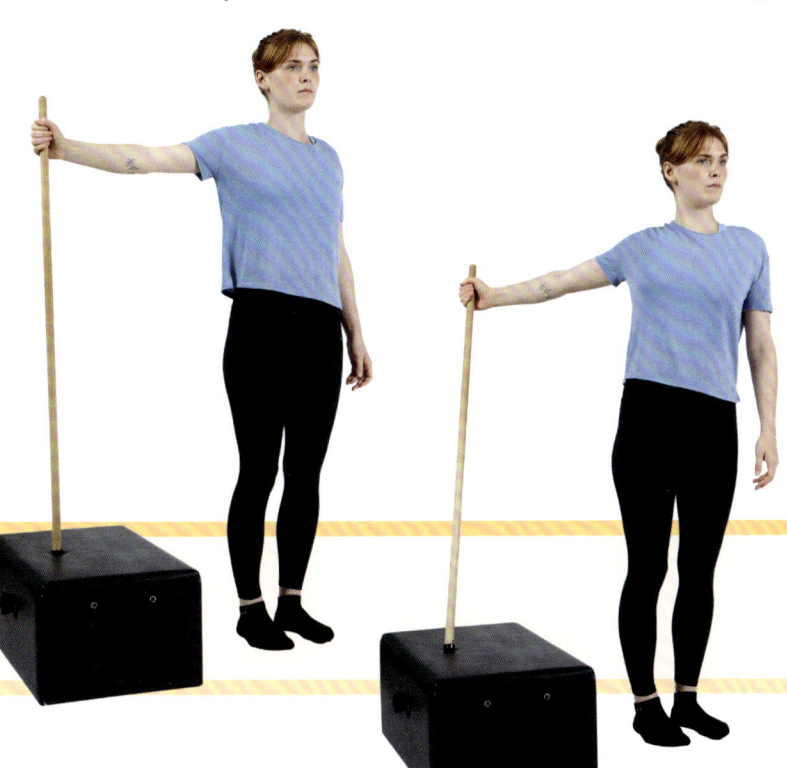

When you reach the end point, this will feel like a one-sided lengthening or pulling in your chest, shoulder and arm. As you repeat the stretch, you should become aware that you are more open and freer in your chest, shoulder and arm.

SELF-MASSAGES

🅡 Spinal muscle massage

Self-massage can be performed before or after the upper back stretches, or at any time to loosen knotted muscles. In this massage, you are unsticking tight muscles between your shoulder blades and spine.

- Stand in neutral posture (*see* p. 35) with your back against a wall.
- Place your massage roller vertically between your spine and your right shoulder blade.
- Lean your body into your roller to get pleasant pressure from it into your muscles.
- Bend and straighten your legs so that the muscles between your shoulder blade and your spine are pulled by the roller.
- The massage roller stays still as your muscles are massaged by it.
- You can also do rolling massage between your shoulder blades and your spine. To do this keep your legs long and gently move your upper back side to side on the roller.
- The movements should be small, and the pressure of the roller into your muscles should be constant.
- Massage for 30-60 seconds.
- Repeat on the left side of the spine.
- **Start with light pressure from your roller into your muscles and if you want to increase the pressure, do so slowly. Avoid putting pressure directly on to your spinal bones or your shoulder blade.**

As you lean in you will feel the pressure of the roller on your back. As you massage you will feel a nudging and pulling sensation in your muscles. As the tightness between the layers of muscles is loosened, you may start to feel warm in the area you're working on.

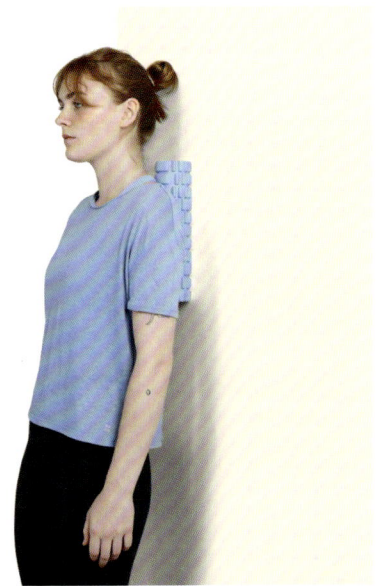

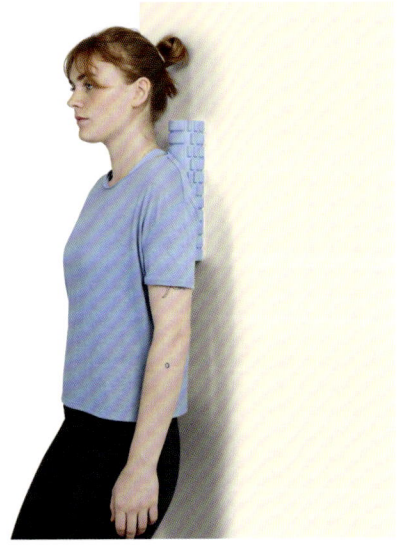

UPPER BACK MOVEMENTS, STRETCHES AND SELF-MASSAGES

ⓡ Upper back massage

When you massage, your muscles get pulled and nudged by the roller. This particular massage involves both a cross-fibre and a rolling action. This helps to loosen tight or knotted muscles and to restore full and free movement to your upper back. This massage is particularly beneficial for people who feel stiff and achy in the upper back in the morning or after a long day at their desk.

- Stand in neutral posture (*see* p. 35) with your back against a wall.
- Place your massage roller horizontally between the wall and your back, just below your shoulder blades. Turn yourself slightly to the right to avoid direct pressure on your spinal bones.
- Lean your body into your roller to get pleasant pressure into your muscles.
- Bend and straighten your legs to roll the massage roller up and down your back muscles, a few centimetres on either side of your starting point.
- You can also do cross-fibre massage in this area. To do this keep your legs long and gently move your upper back side to side on the roller.
- Maintain a consistent gentle to medium pressure on your muscles from your roller.
- Massage for 30-60 seconds.
- Move the roller to higher or lower positions and repeat.
- Change to the left side and repeat.
- **Start with light pressure from your roller into your muscles and if you want to increase the pressure, do so slowly. Don't push too hard and don't bend your knees too deeply – they should come no further forwards than the middle of your foot.**

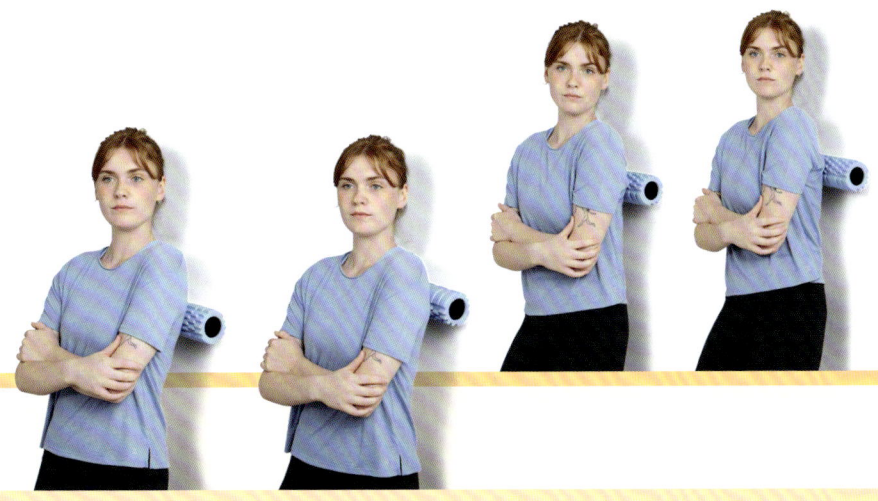

You will feel the pressure of your roller on your back as you lean in. Then as you bend and straighten your legs you will feel a rolling massage sensation in the muscles to one side of your spine. Make sure you avoid rolling over the bony parts of your spine. When you massage it may feel warm in the area you're working on.

MAKE MOVEMENT YOUR MEDICINE

® Side of back massage

This is another self-massage that involves both rolling and cross-fibre actions. This helps to loosen tight or knotted muscles and to restore full and free movement to the upper back and shoulder. This is particularly beneficial to people who work their bodies during the day, such as trades people, gardeners, sports people and carers.

- Stand in neutral posture (*see* p. 35) with your back against a wall.
- Cup the back of your head with your left hand. Alternatively, you can place your left arm across the front of your chest.
- Position your massage roller below and behind your left underarm, below the bottom of your right shoulder blade and across your back. Turn your body slightly to the left side so that the roller is on your muscles rather than the bony rib area.

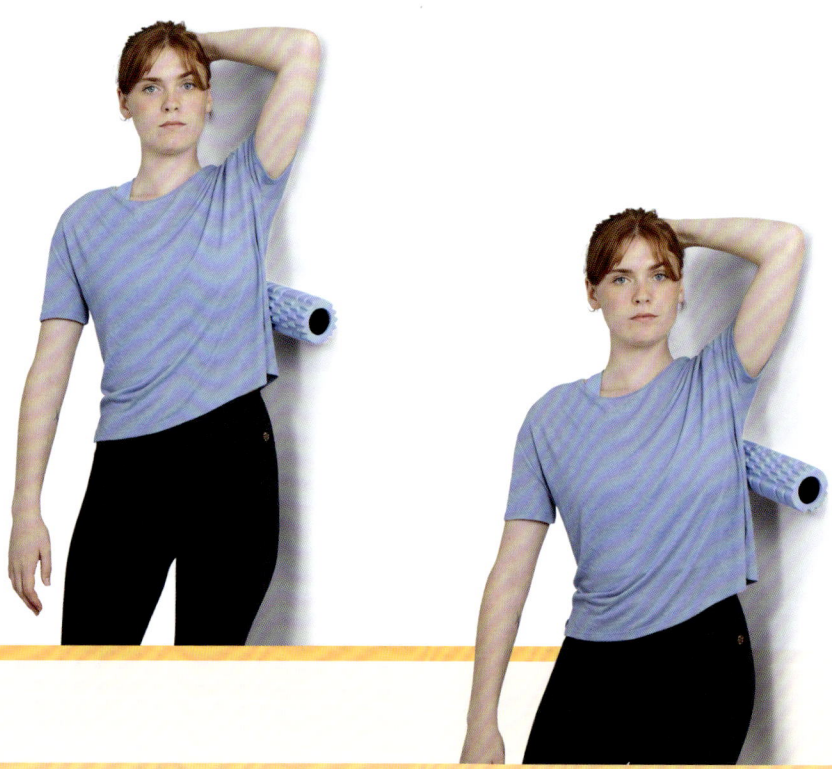

UPPER BACK MOVEMENTS, STRETCHES AND SELF-MASSAGES

You will feel the pressure of your roller on your muscles as you lean in, particularly if you have your hand behind your head, as this will pre-stretch the muscles. Then as you bend and straighten your legs you will feel a rolling massage sensation in the muscles around the bottom of your shoulder blade. Make sure you avoid rolling over the bony parts of your shoulder blade. When you massage it may feel warm in the area you are working on. You should feel it's easier to move your upper back after massaging this area.

- Lean into your roller to apply a pleasant pressure into your muscles.
- Bend and straighten your legs to roll the massage roller up and down a few centimetres on either side of your starting point.
- Roll into the area for 30-60 seconds, focusing on any point that feels tight or knotted.
- To cross-fibre massage this area, keep your legs still and move your body forwards and backwards (left to right and right to left) a few centimetres along your roller. You are pulling or nudging your muscles across your roller, to release stickiness between your muscle layers.
- Massage any point with consistent pressure for 30-60 seconds.
- Change to the right side and repeat.
- **Start with light pressure from the roller into your muscles and increase it if you want a deeper massage. With the cross-fibre massage the roller should not just pull your skin: it should be nudging and moving your muscles at the point you are massaging.**

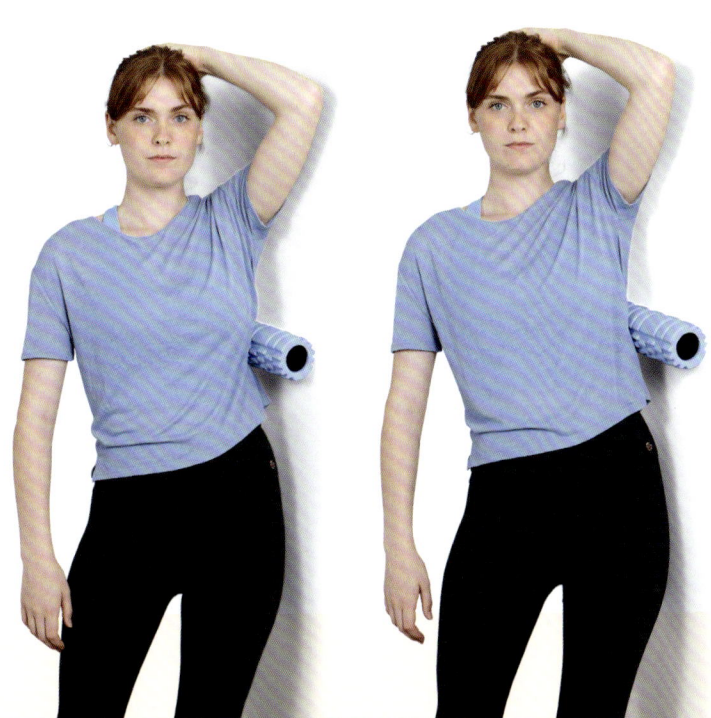

7 NECK MOVEMENTS, STRETCHES AND SELF-MASSAGES

NECK MOVEMENTS, STRETCHES AND SELF-MASSAGES

Our necks are put under immense stress by modern living, and remaining in the same position for extended periods can cause tension and pain. These exercises will help resolve those issues and enable you to keep your neck healthy.

Remember:

- You don't need to do all the movements, stretches and self-massages in this section at once, and you don't have to do them in any particular order.
- Identify the exercises you find most effective and enjoyable or use the tightness tests (*see* pp. 42–53) to identify which you need most and build them into your daily routine.
- It is helpful to start with the three essential upper back exercises (*see* p. 116) as these will help to take strain off your neck.
- It's a good idea to do the neck settling movements (see p. 81) after each stretch to soothe and calm the muscles and joints (you can do these at other times, too).

- All the exercises in this section are designed to keep your neck mobile or, if you have pain in your neck, to make it more comfortable.
- When doing any of these exercises, try to keep your tummy pulled in and – most importantly – don't forget to breathe.
- It is fine to work towards pain, but don't work through it (*see* p. 10). Even if you can work only in a very small, pain-free range, it's still worth doing.
- If your muscles do feel sore or ache from the exercises, it may be helpful to apply heat or a cold pack and gently massage them, as this will help them adjust to healthy movement.

> **EXERCISE SYMBOLS**
>
> To help you identify whether an exercise needs any equipment, we have included a **P** symbol for stretches that require a pole, and an **R** symbol for self-massages that require a roller.

Table 7.1 Neck exercises quick reference

Page number	Movements	Benefits
81	Neck settling movements × 3	Relaxes the neck after the stretches or when the neck has become stiff
82	Turn right, turn left	Releases tightness, helping your head to be able to turn easily
83	Slide the chin in	Releases tightness, helping your head and neck to align into good posture
84	Neck saucer glide	Helps to restore natural movement to your upper neck when it is stiff and achy
Stretches		
85	Back of neck stretch A	Helps to lengthen the back of your neck, releasing tension and restoring good posture
86	Back of neck stretch B	Also helps to lengthen the back of the neck, releases tightness and helps to get rid of a rounded upper back and skin creases in the back of your neck
87	De-stress your neck	A deep stretch to release tightness in the side of your neck and helps improve head, neck and shoulder posture
88	Decompress your neck	Stretches the muscles in the 'back corner' of the neck and reduces neck pain
89	Release your neck	Releases tension in the front and side of your neck, improves forward head posture and helps reduce 'dowager's hump'
Self-massages		
90	Nodding neck massage	Helps to loosen stiff neck muscles so the neck can move more freely
91	Rotating neck massage	Improves rotational movements of the neck
92	Lying down neck massage	Helps you achieve a more comfortable and relaxed neck

NECK MOVEMENTS, STRETCHES AND SELF-MASSAGES

MOVEMENTS

Neck settling movements × 3

Settling movements help to soothe and calm the muscles and joints into their new positions after stretches and are useful reset exercises. Do them between each neck stretch; you can also do them as standalone exercises.

- Stand or sit in neutral posture (*see* p. 35 or p. 38).
- Make sure your head is gently drawn back, with your chin level and your ears over the middle of your shoulders. You will feel the back of your neck lengthening.
- Look at a spot ahead of you.
- Exercise 1: Gently move your head up and down 6–8cm (2–3in) as if you're doing little 'yes' nods. Repeat 3–5 times.
- Exercise 2: Gently turn your head to the right and left, moving 6–8cm (2–3in) each side. This time you are making small 'no' movements. Repeat 3–5 times.
- Exercise 3: Gently move your head as if you're drawing a small circle in the air with the end of your nose. Draw 3–5 clockwise circles and 3–5 anticlockwise circles.
- **Keep your movements small; the aim is to relax your neck.**

You will feel your neck muscles gently lengthening and loosening, and your neck should feel more comfortable and relaxed after the movements.

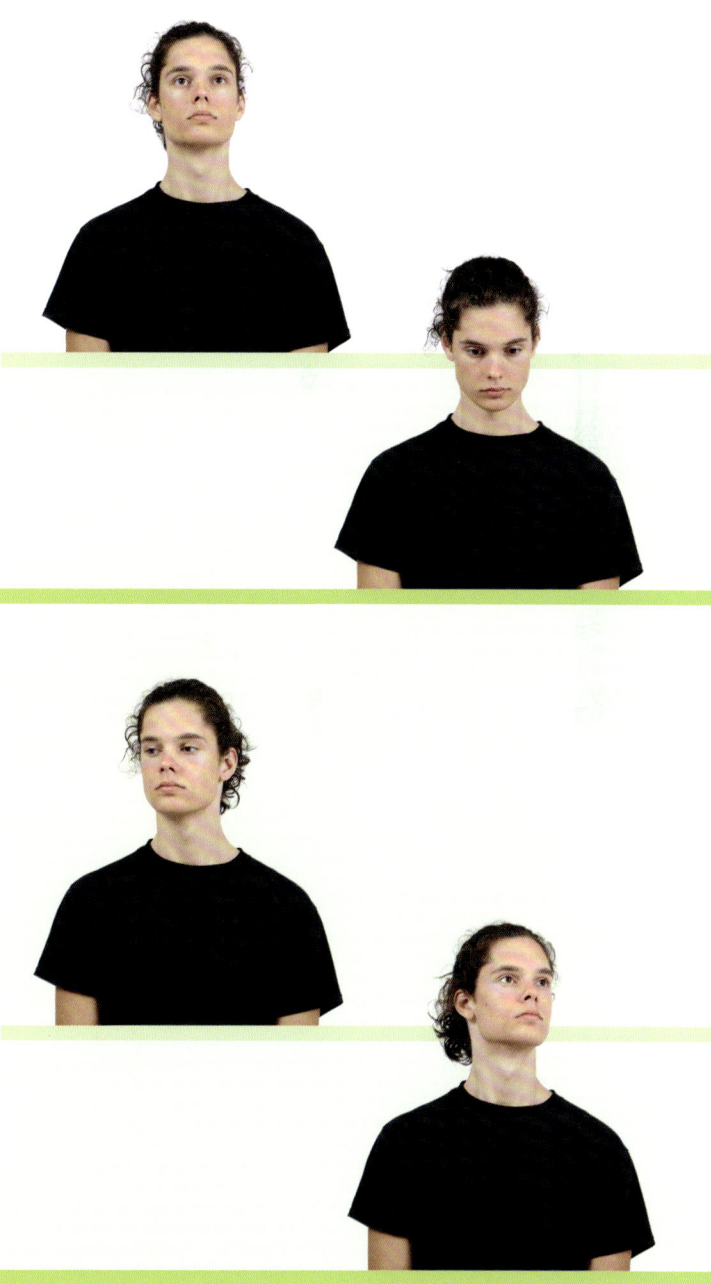

Turn right, turn left

Because we spend so much time with our heads forwards and looking down, we lose the ability to easily turn them. This can increase the chance of straining your neck if you make a sudden movement. This exercise will help release tightness, helping you to turn your head easily.

- Sit in neutral posture (*see* p. 38) on a reasonably firm chair.
- Slowly turn your head to the right as far as you comfortably can, without straining, keeping long through the back of the neck, your chin level and your shoulders down.
- Hold at your end point for 5–10 seconds and remember to keep breathing.
- Come back to the middle and then do the same to the left.
- Repeat 2–5 times letting the movement flow from one side to the other.
- **Make sure you stay in neutral posture. Focus on lengthening the back of your neck and don't force the movement.**

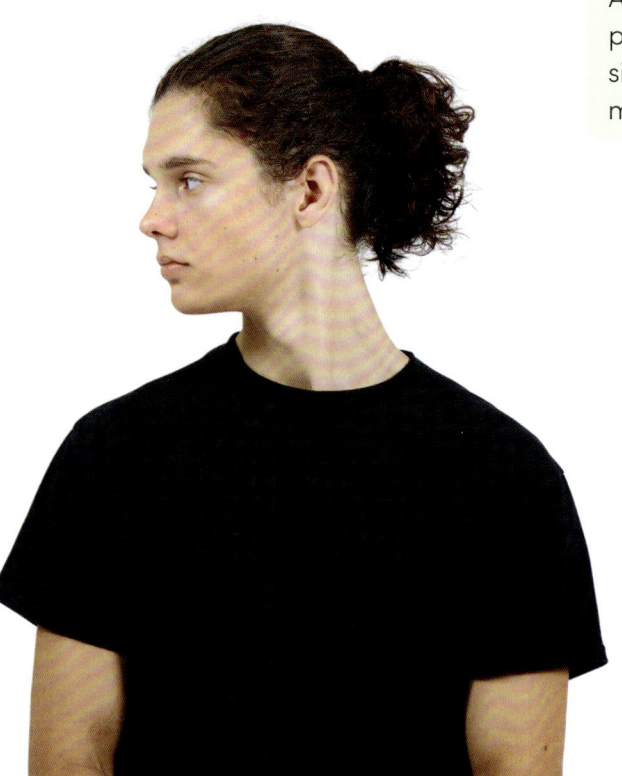

At first you will feel your muscles gently pulling and tightening down one or both sides of the neck, but this sensation will slowly melt away.

Slide the chin in

Modern living can cause our heads to jut forwards, resulting in tightness in the neck. This exercise will release the tightness, helping your head and neck to align.

- Sit in neutral posture (*see* p. 38) on a reasonably firm chair.
- Tuck your elbows into your body, holding your phone or a book level under your chin. The phone or book should have one shorter edge touching your throat.
- Keeping your arms and your phone or book still, gently draw your head back by sliding your chin along the phone or book as far as is comfortably possible.
- Keep your chin in constant contact with the phone or book. The movement is small, slow and smooth, so it might only slide a few centimetres.
- Hold at your end point for a few seconds, then return to the start point.
- Repeat 2–5 times.
- **Make sure you stay in neutral posture. Focus on lengthening the back of your neck and don't force the movement.**

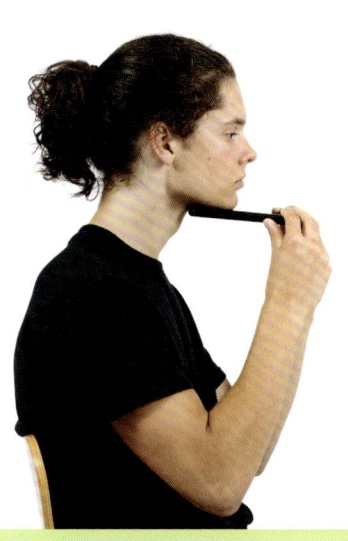
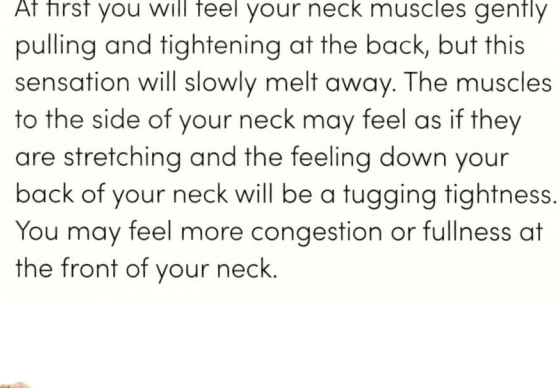

At first you will feel your neck muscles gently pulling and tightening at the back, but this sensation will slowly melt away. The muscles to the side of your neck may feel as if they are stretching and the feeling down your back of your neck will be a tugging tightness. You may feel more congestion or fullness at the front of your neck.

MAKE MOVEMENT YOUR MEDICINE

Neck saucer glide

Sitting slumped with your head forwards can often squash and stiffen the top of your neck. This exercise helps to ease and soothe your upper neck, releasing tension and restoring movement.

- Sit or stand tall in neutral posture (*see* p. 35 or p. 38).
- Gently draw your head back as you lengthen through the back of your neck, aiming to bring your ears over your shoulders.
- Imagine that your head is sitting on a saucer. Start to move your head to the right and at the same time gently lift the right side of your head up, as if it's gliding up towards the right edge of the saucer. The movement is small, slow and smooth.
- Then allow your head to return to the middle of the imaginary saucer before continuing to the left side.
- Repeat 2–5 times as a continuing smooth movement.
- **As you do the movement, think of lifting the back of your ear as your head shifts to the same side. Keep the back of your neck long and do not force the movement.**

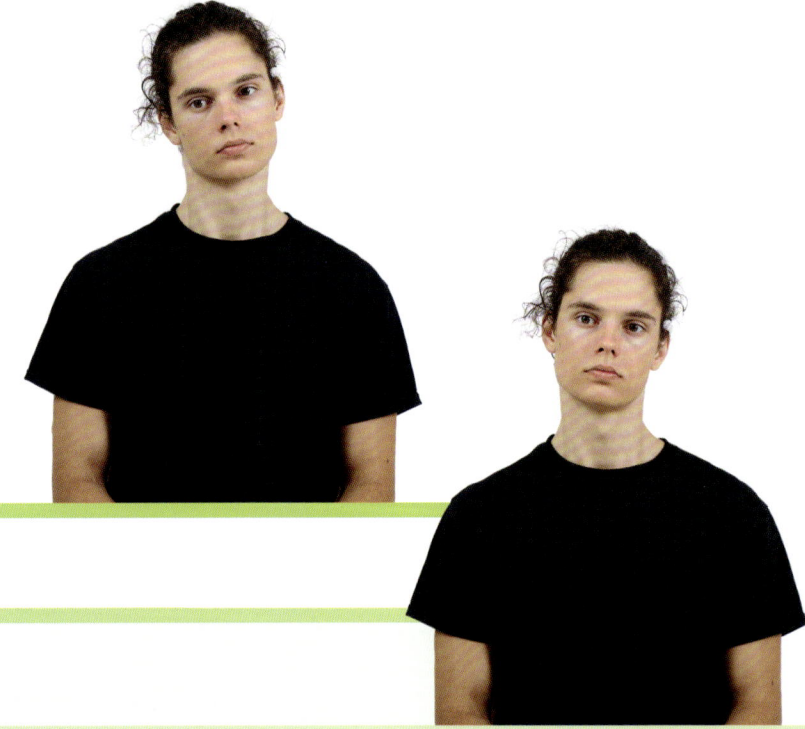

The tightness in your upper neck may feel a little sore and crunchy. This will fade as you do the movement. You will feel a gentle pulling at the side of your neck. You will feel your shoulders and upper back being kept still.

STRETCHES

Back of neck stretch A

This exercise releases tightness in the back of your neck. It also helps to get rid of a 'dowager's hump', rounded upper back and skin creases in the back of your neck. These develop when you slump forwards and your head and chin jut out.

- Sit or stand comfortably in neutral posture (*see* 35 or p. 38).
- Place your fingers on the back of your head, so that they create a barrier for your head to press against.
- Gently push your head back, so that it's pressing into your fingers.
- Let your chin gently lower and try to lengthen the back of your neck.
- Hold this for up to 30 seconds.
- Repeat 2–3 times, doing a few settling movements between each stretch (*see* p. 81).
- **Keep your shoulders relaxed and the pressure of your head pushing into your hand light and consistent.**

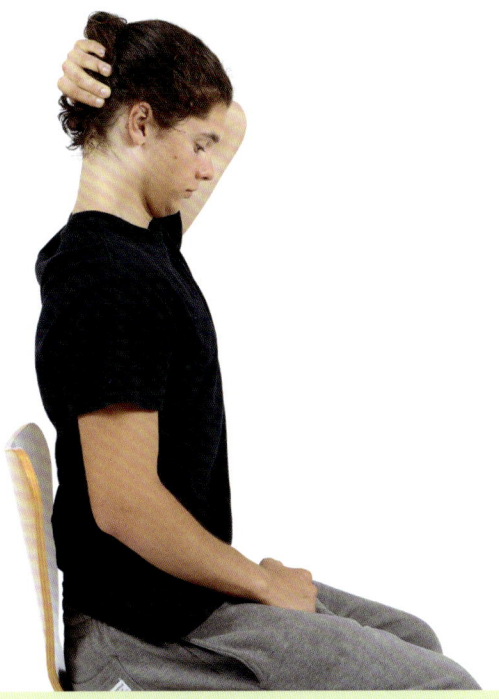

You will feel a stretch in your muscles, which will ease as you hold the stretch and the muscles unstick. When you finish, you may feel lighter and freer in your neck.

Back of neck stretch B

This variation on Back of neck stretch A uses a soft ball or cushion and is done standing, which can be easier on the shoulders. It is a stronger, deeper stretch than the first option.

- Stand tall in neutral posture (see p. 35) against a wall.
- Your feet should be slightly away from the wall and shoulder-width apart. Your back and buttocks should touch the wall. Your arms should be by your side, palms facing forwards.
- Place a soft ball or small cushion behind your head, making sure it doesn't push your head too far forwards.
- Lightly push your head back into the soft ball or cushion, lengthening the back of your neck. Think of trying to slide the back of your head up.
- Add in tiny 'no' movements with your head.
- For a stronger stretch, slowly increase the pressure by pushing your head back harder.
- Do this for up to 30 seconds.
- Repeat 2–3 times, doing settling movements (see p. 81) between each one to relax and settle your muscles into their new lengths.
- **Maintain neutral posture and be careful not to push too hard.**

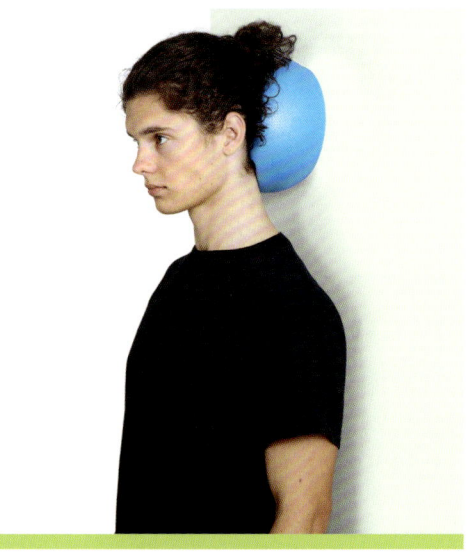

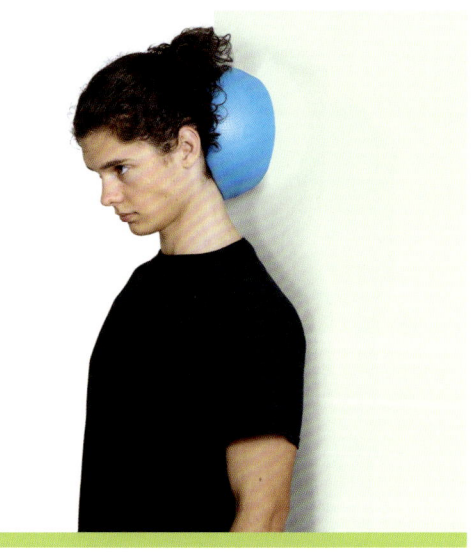

You will feel a tugging stretch in your muscles, but this will ease as you hold the stretch and your muscles unstick. You might feel a fullness or congestion in the front of your neck while doing the stretch, as you will be stretching muscles deep in the front of the neck too. When you finish the stretch you should feel lighter and freer in your neck.

De-stress your neck

Try this stretch if you need to release tightness and discomfort in the side of the neck.

- Sit or stand comfortably in neutral posture (*see* p. 35 or p. 38).
- Keep facing forwards and gently lower your left ear towards your left shoulder. This side is your 'closed' side.
- Bring your left arm over the top of your head and place two fingers on either side of your right ear. This side is your 'open' side.
- Without raising your chin, gently push your head into your fingers, as if lifting your right ear towards where the wall meets the ceiling.
- Hold for up to 30 seconds.
- Repeat 2–3 times on each side, doing a few neck settling movements (*see* p. 81) between each one to relax and settle your muscles into their new lengths.
- **This is only a small movement and you only need to exert a light pressure.**

You will feel a tugging stretch in your muscles, but this will ease as you hold the stretch and your muscles unstick. When you finish the stretch you should feel lighter and freer in your neck.

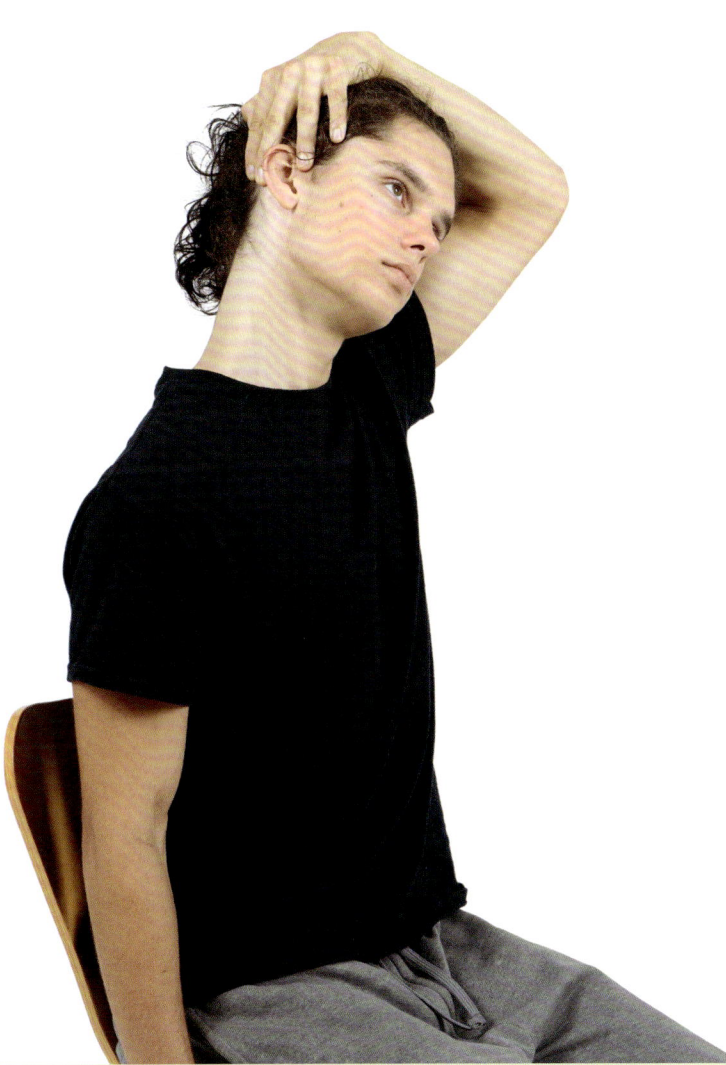

Decompress your neck

The muscles at the back and side of the neck where they meet the shoulder can easily become tight and uncomfortable. This particularly happens when working at a desk or carrying anything heavy, but small movements are enough to stretch the muscles in this area and reduce discomfort.

- Sit or stand comfortably in neutral posture (*see* 35 or p. 38).
- Keep facing forwards as you gently lower your left ear towards your left shoulder. This is your 'closed' side.
- Turn your head slightly to your 'closed' left side.
- Bring your left arm over the top of your head to your right 'open side' and place your fingers just behind your right ear at the base of your skull.
- Relax your 'open side' right shoulder down.
- Gently push your head back against your fingers as if lifting your right ear towards where the wall meets the ceiling.
- Keep your hand and fingers still and feel the light pressure of your head pressing into them.
- Hold for up to 30 seconds.
- Repeat 2–3 times on each side with a couple of settling movements (*see* p. 81) between each one to relax and settle your muscles into their new lengths.
- **Keep the pressure light and the movements small.**

You will feel a tugging stretch in your muscles, but this will ease as you hold the stretch and your muscles unstick. When you finish the stretch you should feel lighter and freer in the side and back of your neck, and the top of your shoulders.

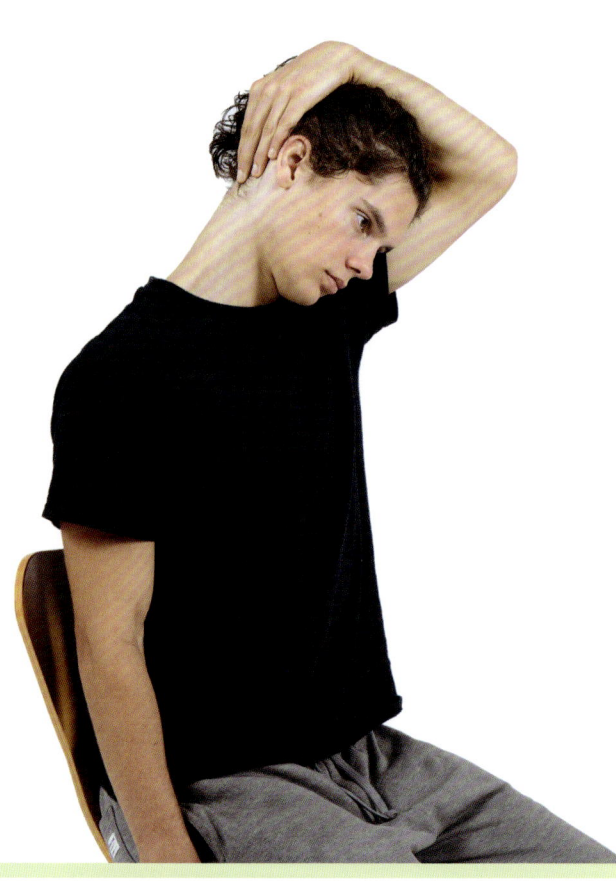

NECK MOVEMENTS, STRETCHES AND SELF-MASSAGES

Release your neck

This exercise specifically helps to release tension in the front and side of your neck, where the muscles often get tight and pull your head forwards. This can particularly affect anyone using screens or phones for work or leisure.

- Sit or stand in neutral posture (*see* 35 or p. 38) with your back supported by the seat or a wall.
- Gently draw your head and neck back and position your ears over your shoulders.
- Take your left hand across your chest and place your fingers on your right collarbone and your palm on your chest.
- Turn your head towards the hand on your collarbone.
- Lower your nose towards your right underarm, still drawing your head back to lengthen your neck.
- Gently lift your skull just behind your right ear on the same side your nose is turned to, while still lowering your nose towards your underarm.
- Hold this position for up to 30 seconds.
- Repeat 2–3 times on each side, doing a few neck settling movements (see p. 81) between each one to relax and settle your muscles into their new lengths.
- **The movements are very small and should be eased into.**

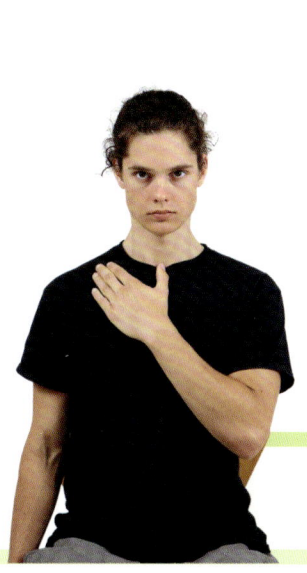
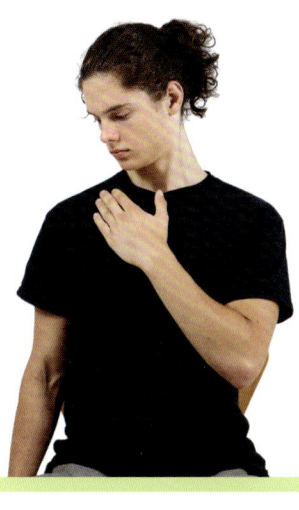

You will feel this mainly in the front, side and slightly in the back of the neck on the side that you are turning your head towards, particularly if you ensure that you keep your head drawn back. The sensation will extend from just above your hand up to the base of your head at the back of your neck and you may even feel it up into your ear. This is fine, as it can even help release excessive tightness in the muscles affecting the ear. You may also feel it on the other side of the neck, but less so if you keep that shoulder relaxed and down. When you finish the stretch you should feel lighter and freer in the side and back of your neck.

SELF-MASSAGES

ⓡ Nodding neck massage

This massage helps to improve the sliding ability of the neck muscles, making it easier to move the neck and achieve a better posture. It is also good for easing tightness in the back and side of the neck.

- Stand with your back and buttocks resting against a smooth wall.
- Place a small cushion behind your head and neck, then place a massage roller between the cushion and your neck. Turn your body slightly to the right.
- Lean into the roller to apply pressure into your neck muscles. Keep the massage roller still and an even pressure on it.
- Lower your chin as though nodding your head.
- Feel the massage roller pulling and moving the muscles to unstick them. Go as far as is comfortable before returning to the start position.
- For a deeper massage, lean into your roller more.
- Repeat 2–5 times on each side.
- **Start with a light pressure and increase it gradually.**

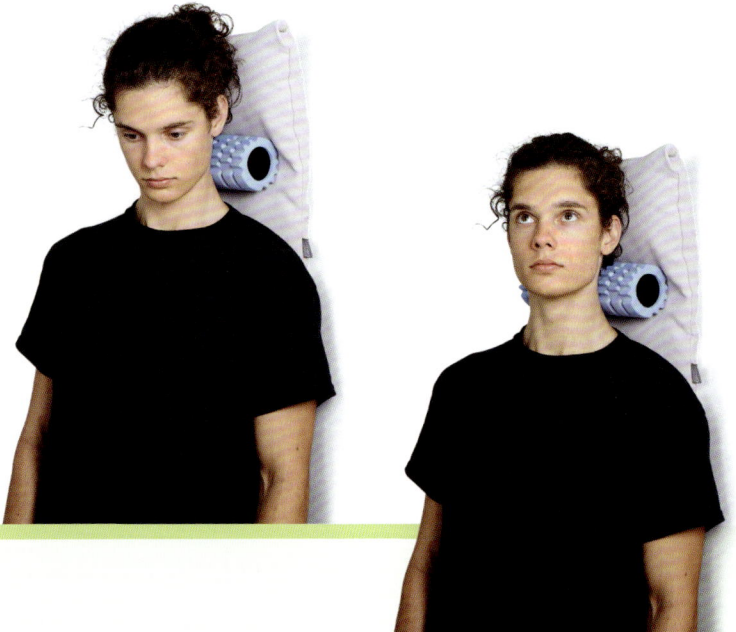

You will feel your neck muscles being kneaded and nudged by the roller. They will feel freer and less tight as you continue with the massage.

NECK MOVEMENTS, STRETCHES AND SELF-MASSAGES

R Rotating neck massage

This has similar benefits to the nodding neck massage, but is especially good for improving rotational movements of the neck.

- Stand with your back and buttocks resting against a smooth wall.
- Place a small cushion behind your head and neck and then place a massage roller between the cushion and your neck.
- Turn your body slightly to the left.
- Lean into the roller to apply pressure into the muscles and lengthen the back of the neck.
- While maintaining an even pressure on the massage roller, which stays still, slowly turn your head to one side. Feel the massage roller squeezing and pulling your muscle layers to unstick them.
- You can lean into the roller for a deeper massage, keeping the back of your neck lengthened.
- Repeat 2–5 times on each side.
- **Start with a light pressure and increase it gradually.**

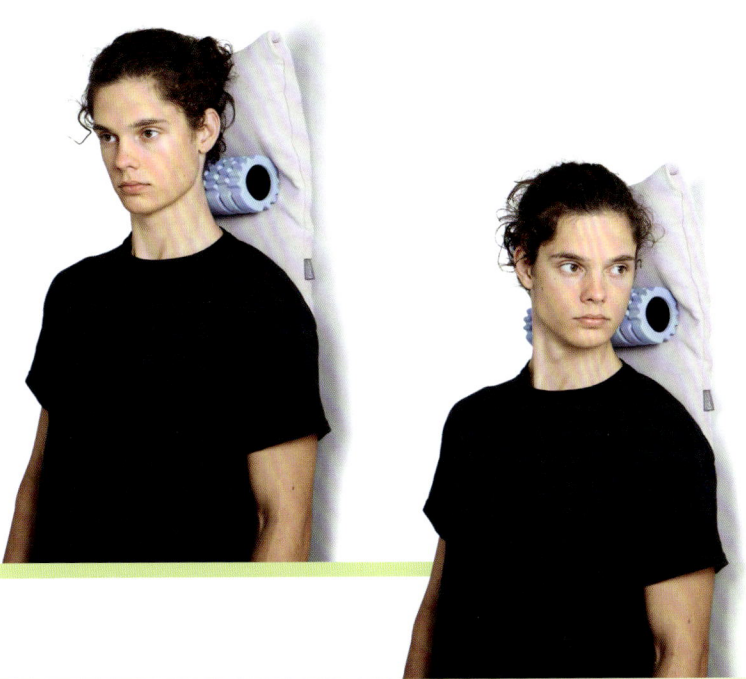

You will feel your neck muscles being kneaded and nudged by the roller. They will feel freer and less tight as you continue with the massage. Your head will turn but the rest of your body will stay still.

🅡 Lying down neck massage

If you have a long-handled massage roller, or a pole with a towel secured around it, this lying down massage method enables you to try a variety of techniques to achieve a more comfortable and relaxed neck.

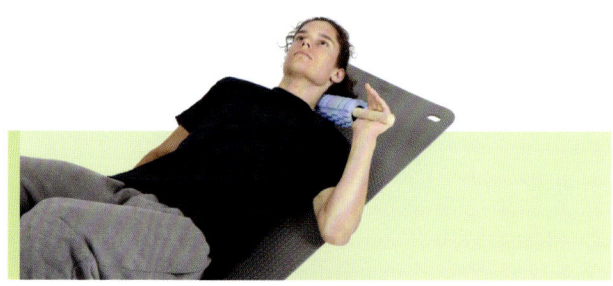

- Lie on your back on a comfortable surface with your knees bent up and feet resting on the floor, hip-width apart.
- Place your massage roller stick behind your neck and hold the end of it with your left hand.
- Keeping your chin tucked slightly towards your chest, lift the end of the roller slightly up off the floor but keep your elbow in contact with the floor.
- Turn your head a little to the left side.
- Keeping your palm open, gently roll the massage roller up and down your left neck muscles.
- Then hold the massage roller still and, keeping your head facing slightly towards the left side, move your head and neck slightly from side to side for a cross-fibre massage.
- Repeat 2–5 times on each side.
- **Keep your neck lengthened. Start with a light pressure and increase it gradually.**

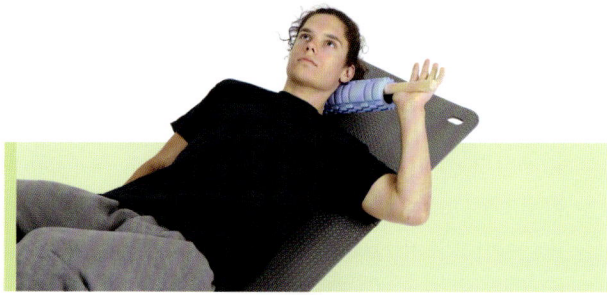

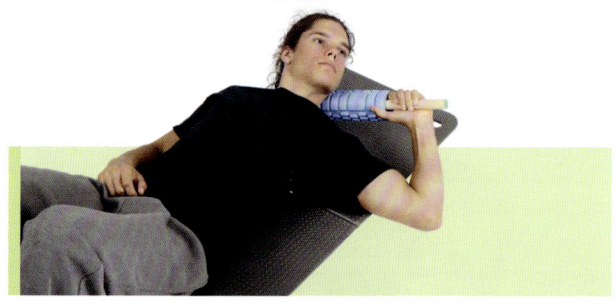

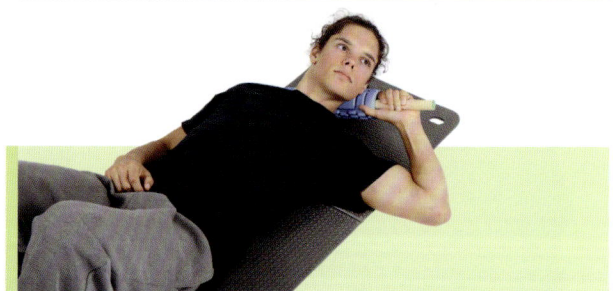

You will feel your neck muscles being kneaded and nudged by the roller. They will feel freer and less tight as you continue with the massage. Your body will stay still as you gently move your head and neck. The muscles in your arm and shoulder will work to hold one end of the roller up and to move it. Keeping the elbow on the floor will help to support the arm.

8 SHOULDER MOVEMENTS, STRETCHES AND SELF-MASSAGES

Your shoulders perform numerous essential tasks and are among the most complicated joints in your body, so you need to look after them. The following exercises will take your shoulders through their full range of movement and help keep them comfortable, supple and injury-free.

- You don't need to do all the movements, stretches and self-massages in this section at once, and you don't have to do them in any particular order.
- Identify the exercises you find most effective and enjoyable or use the tightness tests (see pp. 42–53) to identify which you need most and build them into your daily routine.
- It is helpful to start with the three essential upper back exercises (see p. 116) as these will help to take strain off your shoulders.
- When doing any of these exercises, try to keep your tummy pulled in and – most importantly – don't forget to breathe.
- It is fine to work towards pain, but don't work through it (see p. 10). Even if you can only work in a very small, pain-free range, it's still worth doing.
- If your muscles do feel sore or ache from the exercises, it may be helpful to apply heat or a cold pack and gently massage them, as this will help them adjust to healthy movement.
- Using a pole can often enable restricted shoulders to move by taking and carrying the weight of the arm for the shoulder. If your shoulders are uncomfortable you should also make sure you do at least one hanging stretch (see pp. 104–107), although combining two or more exercises or self-massages will increase the positive effects (see Chapter 9).
- Again, it is a good idea to do the shoulder settling movements (see pp. 96 and 97) after each stretch to soothe and calm the muscles and joints.

> **EXERCISE SYMBOLS**
>
> To help you identify whether an exercise needs any equipment, we have included a **P** symbol for stretches that require a pole, and an **R** symbol for self-massages that require a roller.

SHOULDER MOVEMENTS, STRETCHES AND SELF-MASSAGES

Table 8.1 Shoulder exercises quick reference

Page number	Movements	Benefits
96	Horizontal arm circles (settling movement)	A soothing exercise to maintain relaxed and balanced shoulders
97	Push forward, pull back (settling movement)	Restores and maintains pain-free shoulder movement
98	Pendulum swing front	Improves the range of movement in your shoulders and/or restores pain-free movement
99	Pendulum swing behind	Mobilises your shoulders, making them more relaxed and improving the range of motion
100	Cross-body reach	Keeps your shoulders functioning well and stops them getting tight or stiff
101	Put your coat on	Restores and improves movement in the area of the shoulder you use when putting your arm into a coat
102	Underarm swing	Gently opens your shoulder joint
103	Shoulder blade squeezer	Wakens your shoulder muscles, helping them to function well
Stretches		
104	One-arm forward hang, standing or seated	Opens your shoulder joint, eases tightness in your upper back and restores balance to the shoulder
105	Across-body hang, standing or seated	Stretches and opens up your shoulder joint, easing tightness in the back of the shoulder and down the side of the ribs and the trunk
106	Side hang standing or seated	Stretches and opens up your shoulder joint, and the muscles in and around the shoulder and upper arm and down the side of your body
107	Backward hang	Opens up your shoulder joint, and opens and lengthens the front of the arm, and the front and side of the chest
108	Back scratcher	Restores and improves pain-free reaching behind your back
Self-massages		
109	Shoulder rolling massage	Loosens tight or knotted muscles in the front, side and back of the shoulder to restore full and free movement, which reduces strain on the joint
110	Shoulder cross-fibre massage	Eases restrictions in the fibres of muscles at the front, side and back of the shoulder to restore full and free movement
111	Shoulder blade muscle massage	Loosens tight or knotted muscles at the lower back part of the shoulder to restore full and free movement
112	Top of shoulder massage	Loosens tight or knotted muscles in the top of the shoulder to restore full and free movement, which reduces strain on the joint

MOVEMENTS

Ⓟ Horizontal arm circles

This settling movement uses a pole to soothe and relax the shoulder muscles particularly after a stretch. This helps to avoid cramp and settles the muscles, reducing the risk of strain and injury, as well as making the shoulders feel better in general. You can also do it without a pole, but your shoulder needs to be comfortable taking the weight of your arm.

- Stand comfortably in neutral posture (*see* p. 35) with your feet shoulder-width apart.
- Place a pole vertically in line with your hip and to the side of your body.
- Take hold of your pole with your right hand, holding it at chest height, with your elbow bent.
- Keeping your arm and shoulder relaxed, with the pole taking the weight of your arm, gently move the pole as if stirring a huge cauldron. The end of the pole in contact with the floor should not move.
- Start by moving your bent elbow as far behind you as possible.
- As you make a big circular stirring motion, your arm will naturally straighten as it comes in front of you.
- Bend at the elbow to return to the start position.
- Do this 2–3 times slowly and 2–3 times faster in both clockwise and anticlockwise directions.
- Repeat with the other arm.
- **Keep your shoulders down and your ears above your shoulders, and stay upright, although you might find you rock a little. Only move in a range that is comfortable and without pain.**

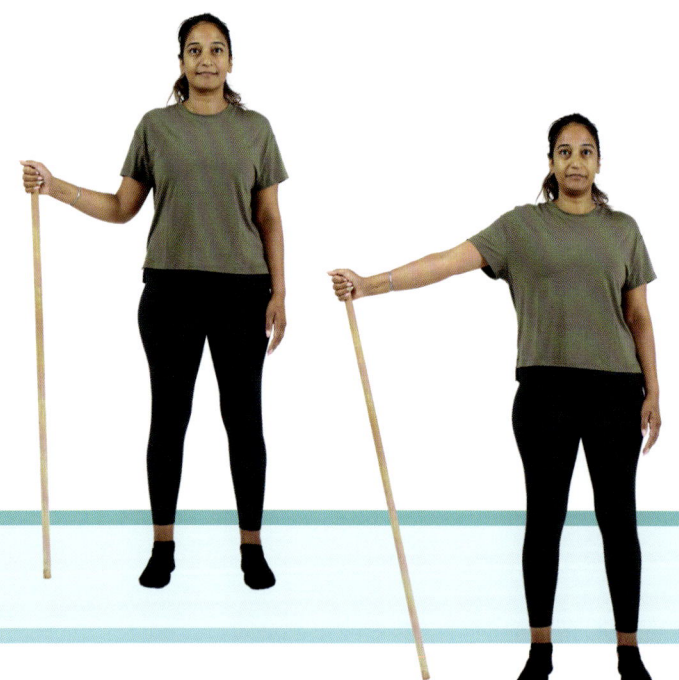

As the pole takes the weight of your arm it will feel like your arm is floating through the movement. You will feel your muscles stretching and this sensation will be a gentle pulling and opening, which will reduce as you continue with the movement. You will feel your shoulder blade squeeze in towards your spine when your elbow bends behind you and relax away from your spine as you lengthen your arm. You will be aware of movement in your shoulder joint and you might feel your chest muscles stretch a little, too.

ⓟ Push forward, pull back

Simple but effective, this settling movement using a pole is a good exercise for restoring and maintaining pain-free shoulder movement, particularly after any shoulder hanging stretches. You can also do it without a pole, but your shoulder needs to be comfortable taking the weight of your arm.

- Stand or sit comfortably in neutral posture (see p. 35 or p. 38) with your feet shoulder-width apart.
- Hold a pole with your right hand at chest height vertically in line with your hip and to the side of your body, with your elbow bent.
- Position your ears over your shoulders but relax your shoulders away from your ears.
- Lengthen your arm forwards as far as is comfortable, then bend your elbow to bring it as far back as possible.
- Keep your hips and legs still. It is natural for your chest to turn gently and for your shoulder to come slightly forwards.
- This is a smooth-flowing continuous motion, going backwards and forwards. Try the movement with your hand at different heights on the pole.
- Repeat the full motion 3–5 times slowly and then 3–5 times faster.
- Swap hands and repeat on the other side.
- **Keep your shoulders down and your ears above your shoulders. Use the pole to guide you and to carry the weight of your arm.**

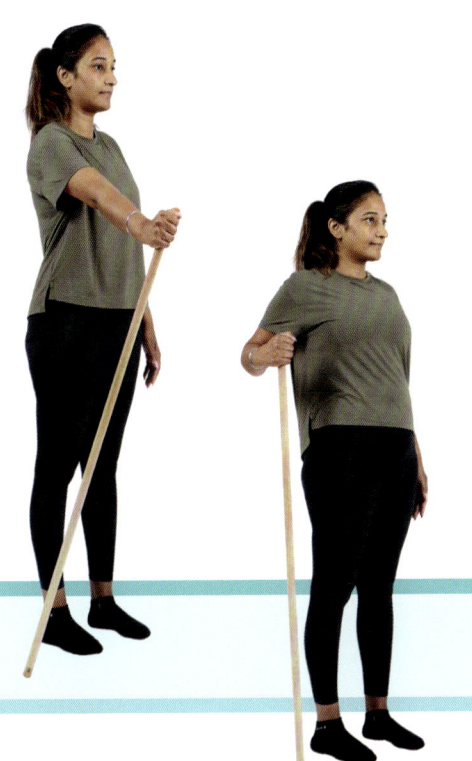

> Stretching can be felt as a tugging sensation in the muscles, which eases as you keep repeating the movement. You will feel your shoulder blade squeeze towards your spine as your elbow bends behind you. You will feel your muscles shorten and lengthen as they create movement.

ⓟ Pendulum swing front

This exercise with a pole is excellent for improving the range of movement in your shoulders and/or restoring pain-free movement.

- Stand in neutral posture (see p. 35) with your feet shoulder-width apart.
- Hold a pole resting in front of your hips with both hands as wide apart as is comfortable.
- Keep your arms fully lengthened, your palms facing your body and your shoulders relaxed down.
- The motion is a smooth swinging one. Lead the movement by lifting the pole as high as possible on one side as the other end lowers. Your arms should stay straight.
- The hand and arm on the side that is lowering will lead the movement, adding as much 'push' as the side that is lifting up needs.
- Swing your pole from side to side continuously like a swing boat. The movement is smooth and a consistent speed.
- Keep your hips, legs and chest still as you move your arms and shoulders in a pain-free range.
- Repeat 3–5 times at a steady pace and then repeat 3–5 times at a faster pace.
- **Keep your shoulders down and your ribs relaxed, so they don't stick out. Stay upright and keep your body still.**

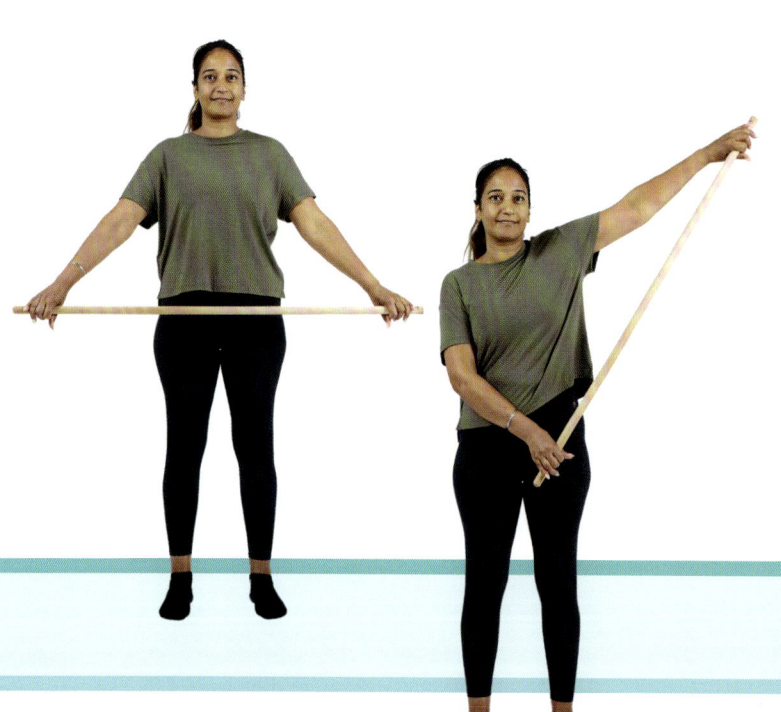

You will feel the muscles on your lead arm, chest and shoulder working to direct and create the movement of the pole swinging. Your arm being pushed up by the pole will feel free and light. As you do the movement your muscles and shoulder joints will feel more open and light. Your tummy, buttocks and leg muscles will gently contract as they work to stabilise you.

SHOULDER MOVEMENTS, STRETCHES AND SELF-MASSAGES

P Pendulum swing behind

This exercise will mobilise and loosen the muscles in your shoulders and ribcage, making them feel more relaxed and improving their range of motion.

- Stand in neutral posture (see p. 35) with your feet shoulder-width apart.
- Hold the pole behind your back with both hands as wide apart as is comfortable. The pole should be horizontal and by your bottom
- Keep your arms straight with your palms facing towards your body and your shoulders open and down.
- The motion is a smooth swinging one. Lead the movement by lifting the pole as high as possible on one side as the other end lowers. Your arms should stay straight.
- The hand and arm on the side that is lowering will lead the movement, adding as much 'push' as the side that is lifting up needs.
- Swing the pole from side to side continuously and smoothly, in a comfortable range. Your hips, legs and chest should stay still. Only your arms and shoulders should move.
- Repeat 3–5 times slowly and then 3–5 times faster.
- **Keep your shoulders down and your ears over your shoulders. Stay upright and keep your body still.**

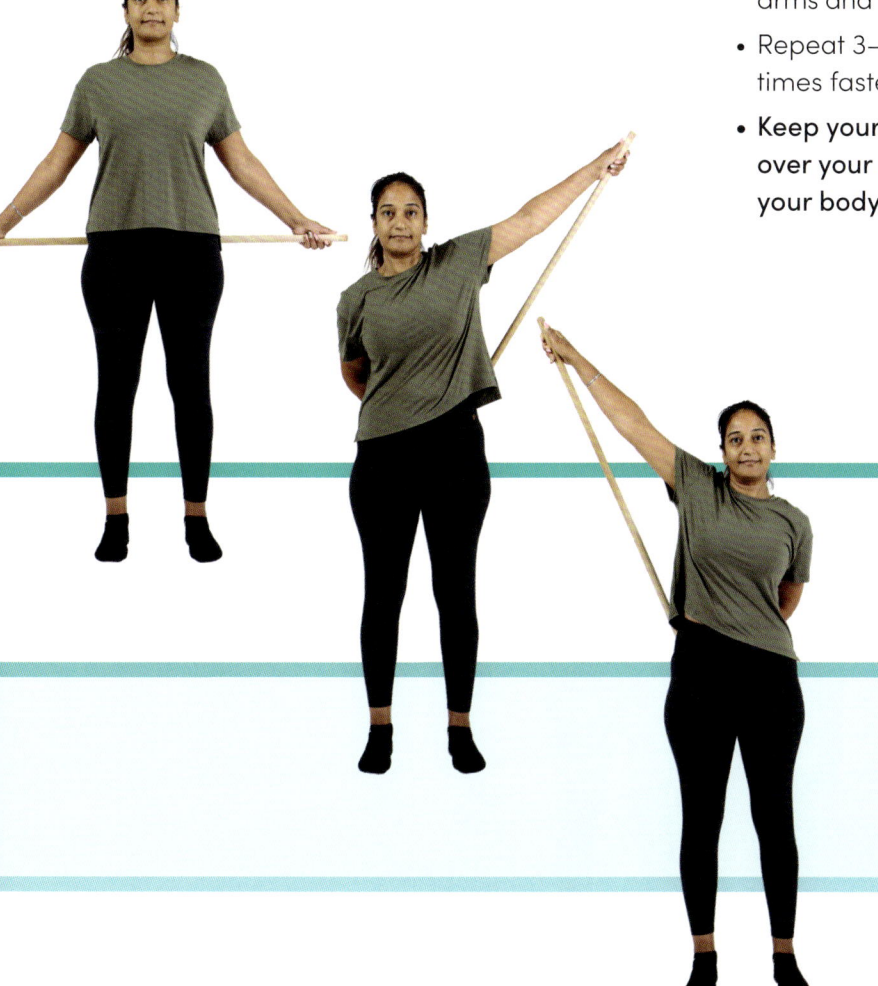

You will feel the shoulder and arm muscles of the pushing arm gradually tightening as the opposite side is pushed further up. You will also feel a gentle stretching in the shoulder, arm and side of the ribcage of the side that is lifting, and a slight squeezing between your shoulder blades. As you continue with the smooth movements your muscles and shoulder joints will feel freer and lighter. You will feel your tummy and buttocks muscles gently working to stabilise you.

P Cross-body reach

This movement helps keep your shoulders functioning well and stops them getting tight or stiff. The pole enables the weight of the arm to be carried, helping the shoulder to move freely.

- Stand in neutral posture (*see* p. 35) with your feet shoulder-width apart.
- Position the pole between your feet, about 15cm (6in) in front with one end on the floor. Hold it at about chest height with your right hand. Bend your elbow and keep your shoulders down.
- Keep your hips and legs still but lengthen your pole arm out to the right-hand side, taking it as far as is comfortable.
- Bring your arm back through the start position and lengthen your pole arm across your body. Your chest will turn a little.
- Let your arm flow smoothly.
- Repeat 3–5 times slowly, then 3–5 times faster on each side.
- **Use the pole to guide you and carry the weight of your arm. Keep upright and still, with your shoulders down and your ears above your shoulders.**

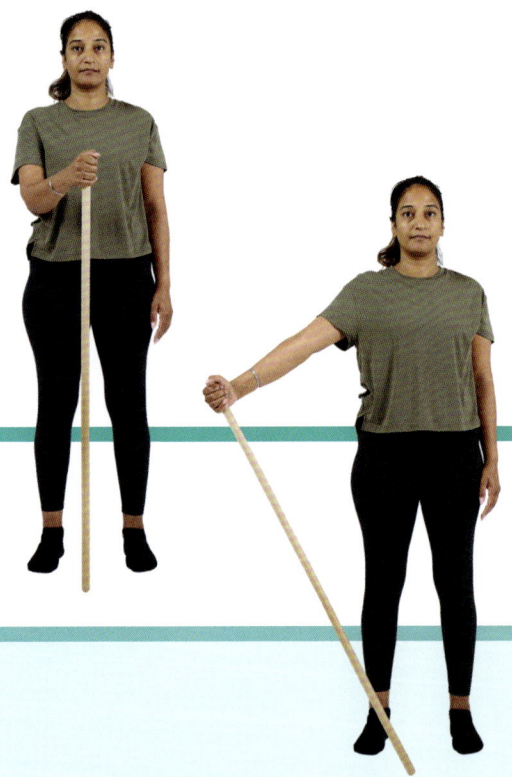

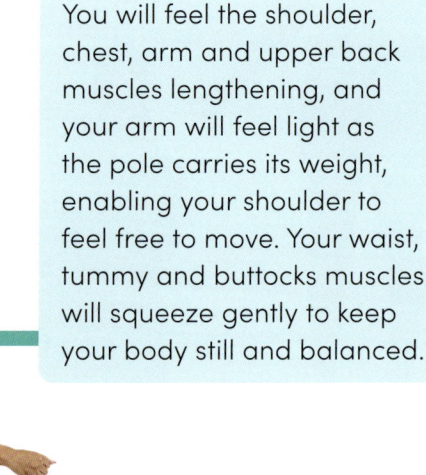

You will feel the shoulder, chest, arm and upper back muscles lengthening, and your arm will feel light as the pole carries its weight, enabling your shoulder to feel free to move. Your waist, tummy and buttocks muscles will squeeze gently to keep your body still and balanced.

SHOULDER MOVEMENTS, STRETCHES AND SELF-MASSAGES

P Put your coat on

This one helps to restore and improve the movement you need in your shoulder when putting your arm into a coat. This is a movement that often becomes difficult when your shoulders start to round and tighten. You can use a pole or broom handle to take the weight of the arm in order to make the shoulder more comfortable but you can also do it without a pole.

- Stand comfortably in neutral posture (see p. 35) with your feet hip-width apart.
- Place a pole vertically about 15cm (6in) out to the side of your right foot and hold it with your right hand at waist level. Your elbow should be bent and tucked into your side. The end of the pole stays in contact with the floor.
- Keeping your elbow bent, move your arm back until your wrist reaches your side. Then fully lengthen your arm behind you.
- Keeping your movement smooth and continuous, swoop your lengthened arm forwards until it is directly in front of your shoulder.
- Bend your elbow again, to return to the start position.
- Keep your hips and chest still and only move your arms and shoulders in a range that is comfortable.
- Repeat 2–5 times on one side and then repeat on the other side.
- **Keep your shoulders down and your ears over your shoulders. Use the pole to guide you, letting it carry the weight of your arm.**

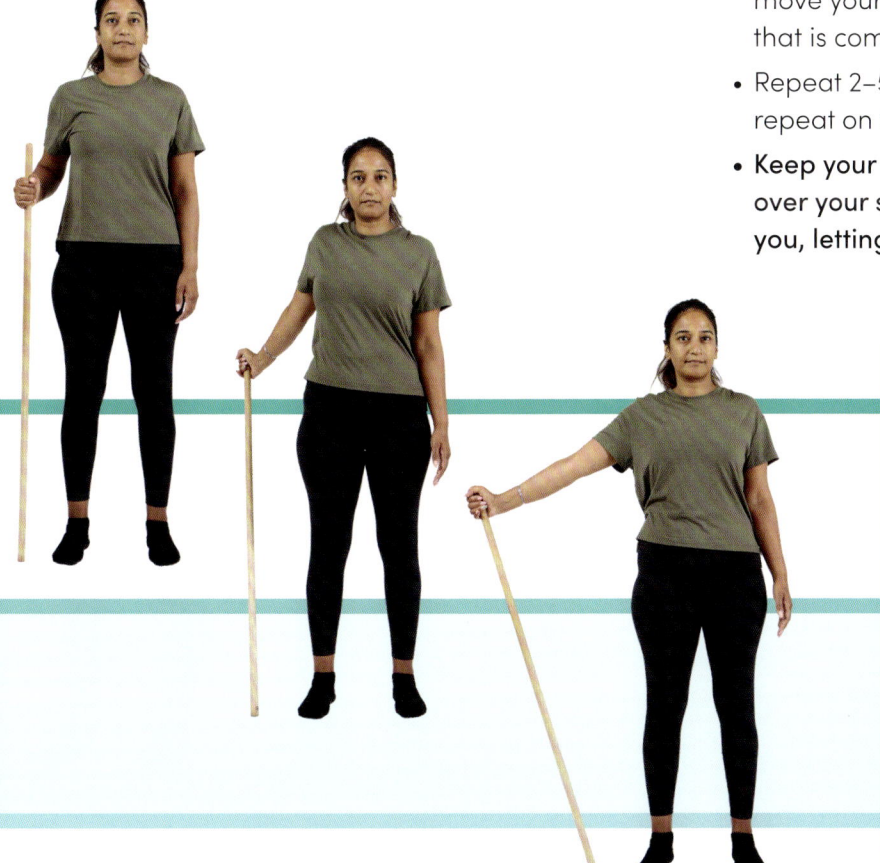

Around the back of your shoulder, your arm and in your upper back you will feel a pulling sensation as the muscles work to do the exercise, but this will melt away as the movement unsticks your muscles. Grip the pole gently to support the weight of your arm, which will feel as if it is floating through the movement. As you repeat this exercise, you will feel your shoulder joint becoming freer.

MAKE MOVEMENT YOUR MEDICINE

ⓟ Underarm swing

This exercise is designed to provide gentle traction to open your shoulder joint, helping it to stay pain free. You need a short pole, but if you don't have one you could use a plastic or metal bottle of water, a tennis racket or something similar.

- Stand comfortably in neutral posture (*see* p. 35) with your feet hip-width apart but with your right foot behind you.
- Hold your pole or chosen item at chest height in your right hand, keeping your shoulders relaxed and down.
- Gently swing your arm backwards, keeping your elbow straight but not over-extended.
- Allow your body to gently rock in rhythm with the pole-swinging movement but keep your hips facing forwards. Your chest will naturally turn a little with the movement.
- Try to keep the movement flowing smoothly through the entire exercise.
- Repeat the movement five times on each side. Don't forget to adjust your feet when you change sides.
- **Keep your shoulders down, your ears above your shoulders and your chin level. Try not to grip the pole too tightly.**

As your arm swings, you will feel an opening or gentle pulling in your shoulder joint and muscles. Your legs, tummy and buttocks will tighten gently to keep you balanced.

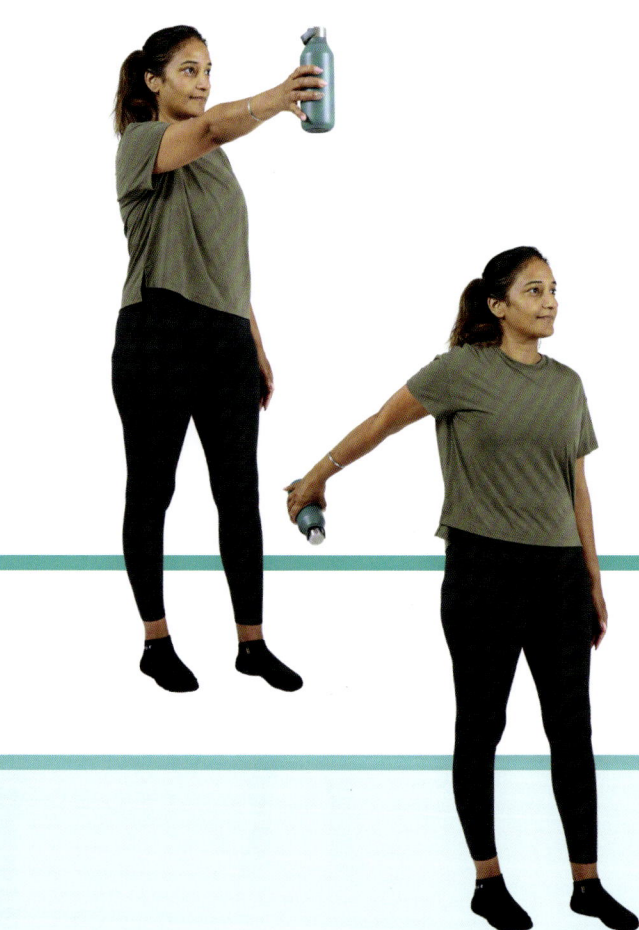

Shoulder blade squeezer

This exercise helps to activate the muscles around your shoulder blades, enabling them to function well.

- Stand or sit in neutral posture (*see* p. 35 or p. 38) with your feet hip-width apart. Keep your ribs and your shoulders relaxed down.
- Bend your arms and tuck your elbows into your side with your forearms parallel to the floor.
- Gently draw your elbows backwards as far as possible.
- Squeeze your shoulder blades together and draw them down your back a little.
- Hold for a couple of seconds and then return to the start position.
- Repeat 2–5 times.
- **Keep your shoulders down, your ears over your shoulders and your ribs relaxed, so they don't stick out. Keep your body still.**

You will feel tightness between your shoulder blades, your back muscles working as your shoulder blades squeeze together, and a stretch in your chest, which will feel like a gentle pulling.

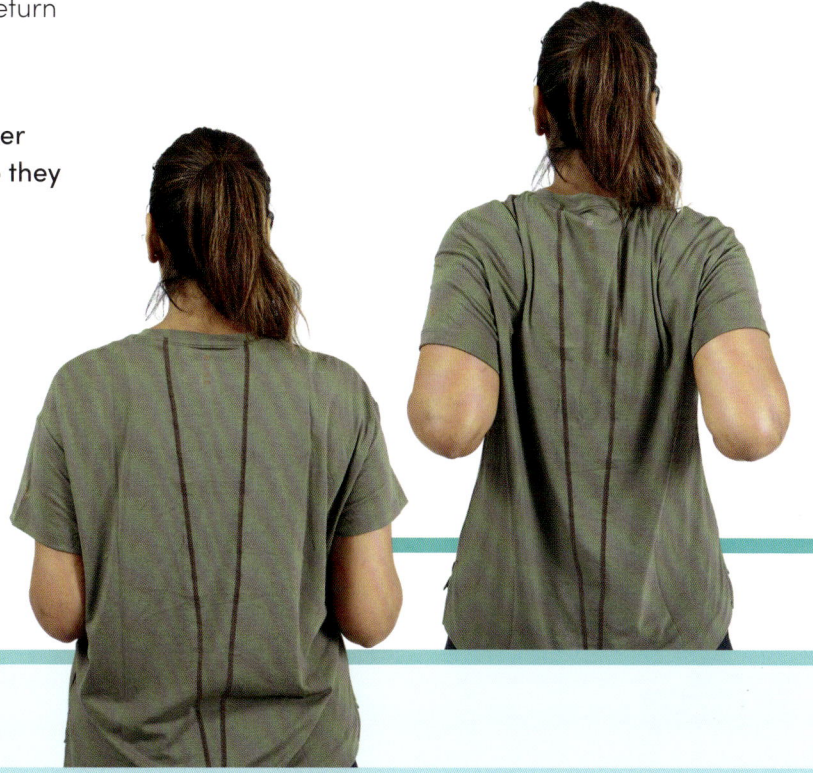

STRETCHES

ⓟ One-arm forward hang, standing or seated

- Sit in a neutral posture (*see* p. 38) with your feet hip-width apart.
- Place a pole vertically out to the right side, in line with your heel.
- Hold the pole with your right hand as high as you comfortably can, keeping your arm straight but relaxed.
- Lean forwards with your back in neutral, pushing the top of the pole out in front of you as far as you can. Keep your arm straight and partly hang on the pole. Think of your underarm opening and lowering towards the base of the pole.
- Gently activate your muscles as if you are going to draw your shoulder blade and underarm towards your back hip. It will feel like you are pulling down on the pole.
- Hold for up to 30 seconds, making sure you breathe, and then return to the start position. If you feel any pinching pain in the top of your shoulder, hold the pole lower down.
- Repeat three times on each side. Do Horizontal arm circles (*see* p. 96) or push Forward, pull back (*see* p. 97) after each stretch to relax and settle your muscles into their new lengths.
- **Try to keep your ears over your shoulders, your feet evenly weighted and your hips square.**

Standing variation

This stretch helps to open the shoulder joint and muscles, as well as the upper back. This exercise is beneficial for anyone who wants good posture and comfortable shoulders.

- Stand tall in neutral posture (*see* p. 35) with your feet hip-width apart.
- Place a pole vertically in front of you on the floor or on a raised surface for the pole to be higher. Make sure the pole is in line with your right shoulder. Hold it with your right hand as high as you comfortably can, keeping your arm straight but relaxed.
- Slowly bend your knees and stick your buttocks out as if lowering into a chair. Keep your arm straight and partly hang on the pole. Think of your underarm gently opening towards the base of the pole.
- The rest of the movement is as described on the left for sitting.

> As you lean into the hanging stretch, you will feel a gradual lengthening of the arm, an opening of the shoulder, and a lengthening stretch of the upper back muscles from the shoulder to the lower ribs on the side that you are stretching.

SHOULDER MOVEMENTS, STRETCHES AND SELF-MASSAGES

(P) Across-body hang, standing or seated

This movement helps to stretch and open up the shoulder joint. It is particularly good for easing tightness in the back of the shoulder and down the side of the ribs and the upper back.

- Stand tall in neutral posture (*see* p. 35) with your feet shoulder-width apart.
- Place a pole vertically in front of you, in between and slightly in front of your feet, with one end on the floor or on a raised surface for the pole to be higher. Hold it with your right hand as high as you comfortably can, keeping your arm straight but relaxed.
- Bend your knees and stick your buttocks out, as if to lower yourself into a chair. At the same time, reach the pole across your body, keep your arm straight, and partly hang on the pole. You can also turn your head and chest slightly towards the pole.
- Try to activate your muscles gently to draw your shoulder and underarm towards your hip. It will feel as if you are gently pulling down on your pole.
- Hold for up to 30 seconds while breathing and then slowly return to the start position.
- Repeat three times on each side. Do horizontal arm circles (*see* p. 96) or push forward, pull back (*see* p 97) after each hanging stretch to help to settle and relax your muscles to their new lengths.
- Try to keep your ears over your shoulders, your feet evenly weighted and your hips square.

Seated variation

- To do this exercise while seated, sit in a neutral posture (*see* p. 38) with your feet shoulder-width apart.
- Place a pole vertically between your feet.
- Hold the pole with your right hand as high as you comfortably can, keeping your arm straight but relaxed.
- The rest of the movement is as described left, for standing.

In this stretch your arm, shoulder and back muscles will feel a tightening and tugging sensation. You will feel an opening in your shoulder as you enter and hold the hanging stretch. Through your underarm and back you will feel a widening, lengthening or gentle pulling sensation. You might be aware of your muscles working around your shoulder blade. Your tummy and buttocks muscles will contract to keep your lower body still.

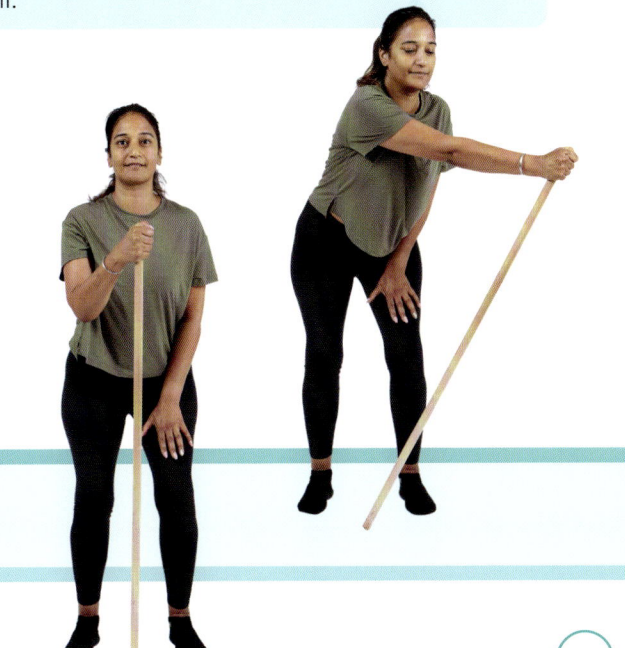

🅟 Side hang, standing or seated

The side hang helps to stretch and open up the shoulder joint. It also stretches the shoulder muscles and upper back. It might also stretch down the side and slightly into the front of your body.

- Stand tall in neutral posture (*see* p. 35) with your feet shoulder-width apart.
- Place a pole vertically out to the right side of you in line with your toes, with one end on the floor or on a raised surface for the pole to be higher.
- Slowly bend your knees and stick your buttocks out, as if to lower yourself into a chair.
- Keep your arm straight as you lean into a gentle hang, pushing the pole further out to the side.
- Try to get your muscles to gently activate, as if to draw your shoulder and underarm towards your hip.
- Hold for up to 30 seconds and then slowly return to the start position.
- Repeat three times on each side. Do horizontal arm circles (*see* p. 96) or push forward, pull back (*see* p. 97) after each hanging stretch to help to settle and relax your muscles at their new lengths.
- **Try to keep your ears over your shoulders, your feet evenly weighted and your hips square.**

• Seated variation

- To do this exercise while seated, sit in a neutral posture (*see* p. 38) with your feet shoulder-width apart.
- Place a pole vertically out to the right, in line with the front of the chair.
- Hold the pole with your right hand as high as you comfortably can, keeping your arm straight but relaxed.
- The rest of the movement is as described left, for standing.

> As your arm, shoulder and back stretch you will feel a tightening or tugging sensation in the muscles as they lengthen. You will feel an opening sensation in your shoulder as you do the hanging stretch. Through and around your underarm you will also feel an opening, lengthening or gentle pulling sensation. You might be aware of the muscles around your shoulder blade on the pole side, working to stabilise it. Your tummy and buttocks muscles will contract to keep your lower body still.

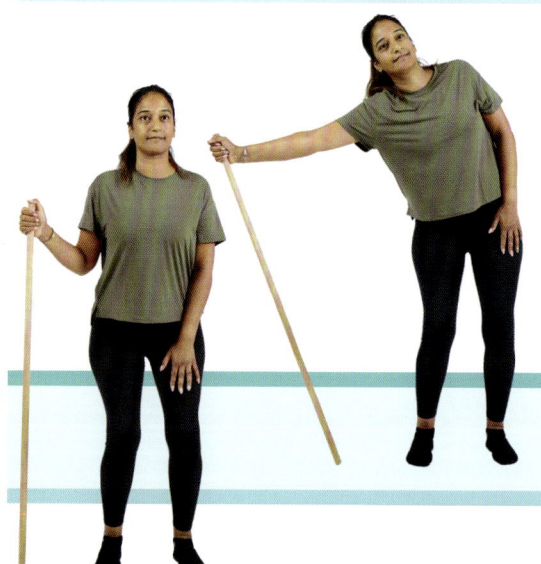

SHOULDER MOVEMENTS, STRETCHES AND SELF-MASSAGES

Ⓟ Backward hang

This hanging back stretch is a particularly strong stretch, so go into it slowly and gently. It helps to open up the front of the shoulder joint and will also open and lengthen the front of the arm, and the front and side of the chest. This one is especially good for tennis players and swimmers.

- Stand tall in neutral posture (*see* p. 35) with your feet shoulder-width apart.
- Place a pole vertically in line with your right heel and out to the side. Hold it with your right hand as high as you comfortably can, on a raised surface if needed. Your arm should be straight, but not over-extended at your elbow.
- Slowly bend your knees and stick your buttocks out, as if to lower yourself into a chair.
- At the same time, gently angle the top of the pole behind you.
- Keep your arm straight as you lean into a gentle shoulder hang.
- Try to gently activate your muscles as if to draw your shoulder and underarm down to your hip.
- Hold for up to 30 seconds and then slowly return to the start position.
- Do horizontal arm circles (*see* p. 96) or push forward, pull back (*see* p. 97) after each hanging stretch to settle your muscles to their new lengths.
- Repeat 1–3 times on each side.
- **Try to keep your ears over your shoulders, your feet evenly weighted and your hips square. Keep the back of your neck long, with your chest and head facing forwards.**

As your arm, shoulder, chest and back stretch you will feel a tightening or pulling sensation in the muscles as they lengthen. You will feel an opening sensation as your shoulder enters and holds the hanging position. Through and around your underarm you will feel an opening, lengthening or gentle pulling sensation. You might be aware of your shoulder blade drawing down to stabilise your shoulder. Your tummy and buttocks muscles will contract as they support your lower body.

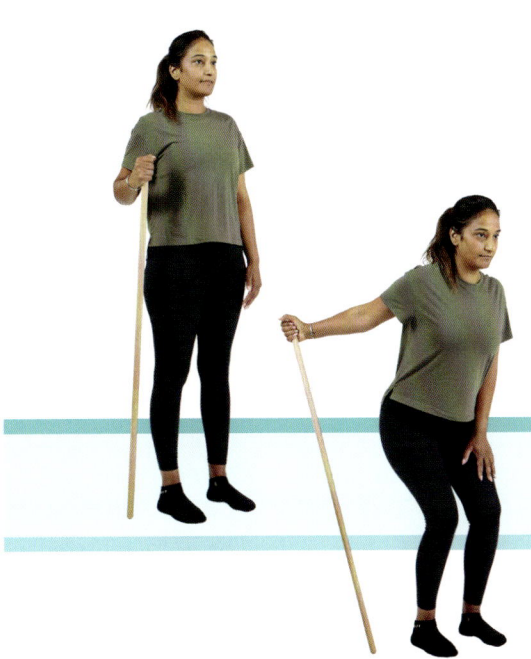

MAKE MOVEMENT YOUR MEDICINE

ⓟ Back scratcher

This stretch will restore and improve pain-free reaching behind your back. You need this movement to scratch your own back or do up a back zip.

- Stand in neutral posture (*see* p. 35) with your feet shoulder-width apart and your right side side-on to a wall, but away from the wall. Keep your shoulders relaxed.
- Place the bottom of a pole against the base of the wall to stop it slipping. Hold it with your right hand behind your lower back with your palm out.
- Slowly take tiny sideways steps towards the wall so that, as you move, your right hand naturally slides up your back. Keep taking tiny steps until you reach your natural end point.
- Let your shoulder relax and widen across the front.
- Hold for up to 30 seconds, breathing and relaxing to unstick any tightness. Then slowly return to the start position.
- Repeat 1–3 times on each side. Do horizontal arm circles (*see* p. 96) or push forward, pull back (*see* p. 97) after each hanging stretch to relax and settle your muscles into their new lengths.
- **Keep upright and still, with your shoulders down and your ears above your shoulders. Use the pole to guide you and to carry the weight of your arm. It is normal to feel tightness in your muscles but only move in a range that is pain free.**

> You will feel a pulling in and around the shoulder as it stretches and opens. You might feel a gentle squashing in the muscles around your shoulder blade and in your back as your hand slides up your back. You want to feel your shoulders widening, opening and relaxing across the front. Your leg, tummy and buttocks muscles will grip gently to stabilise your lower body.

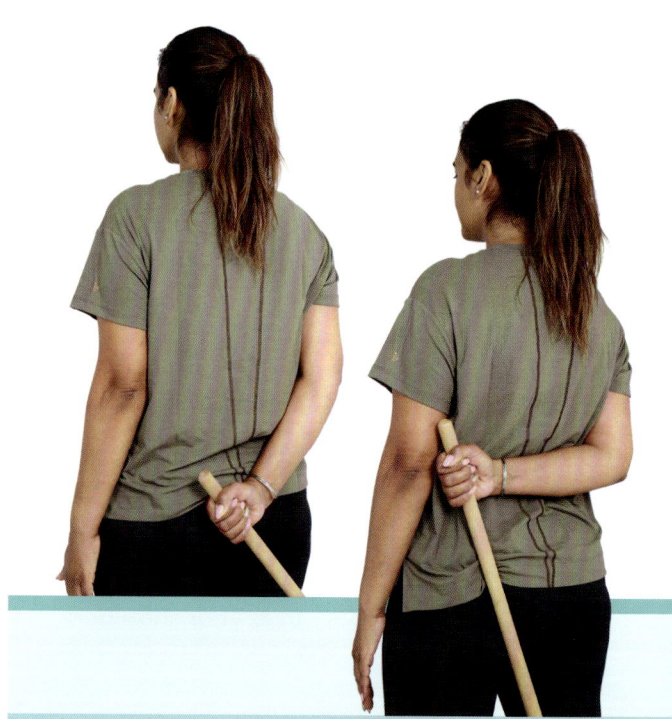

SHOULDER MOVEMENTS, STRETCHES AND SELF-MASSAGES

SELF-MASSAGES

R Shoulder rolling massage

This is a simple self-massage technique that helps to loosen tight or knotted muscles and to restore comfort and full and free movement, which reduces strain on the joint. It can be done on all parts of the shoulder: start on the side of your shoulder and upper arm, then work round to the front and back of your shoulder muscles.

- Stand in neutral posture (*see* p. 35) with the side of your left shoulder or upper arm close to a smooth wall.
- Place your massage roller horizontally between the wall and the side of your shoulder or upper arm.
- Gently lean in towards the wall and the roller to apply a gentle, consistent pressure into your muscles. from the roller.
- Bend and straighten your legs to roll the roller up and down a few centimetres on either side of the start position.
- Massage around the front and back of the shoulder and upper arm by turning your body slightly away from the wall or in towards the wall.
- Roll into any area for up to 30 seconds, focusing on areas that feel restricted, tight or knotted.
- Repeat with your right shoulder.
- **As you begin to roll up and down, you may find some areas are a little knotted and uncomfortable, so don't press too hard at first.**

As you repeat the massaging action the muscles will start to soften, feel freer and more comfortable. This is particularly realised when you return to the massage on subsequent days.

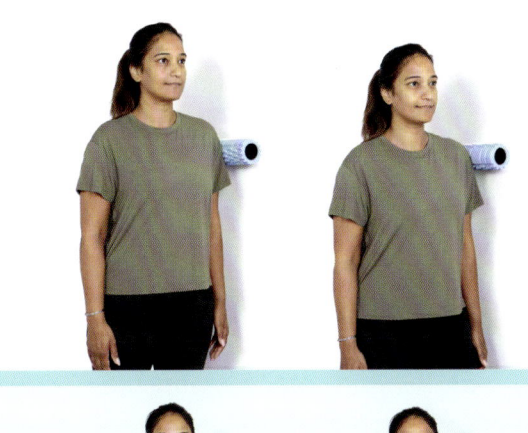

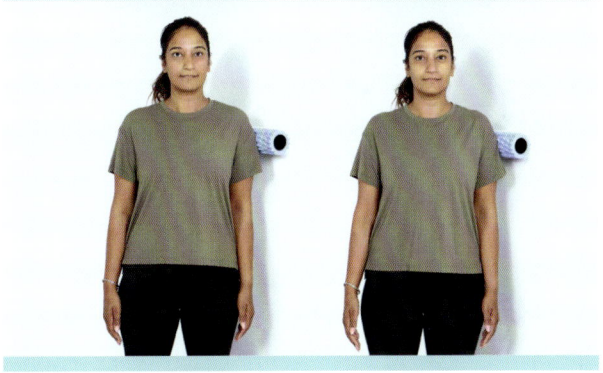

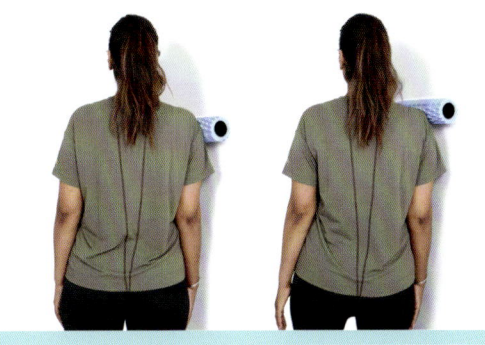

Ⓡ Shoulder cross-fibre massage

This simple self-massage technique helps to loosen tight or knotted muscles and to restore full comfort and free movement to the shoulder muscles which reduces strain on the joint.

- Stand in neutral posture (*see* p. 35) with the side of your left shoulder or upper arm close to a smooth wall.
- Place a massage roller horizontally between the wall and the part of your shoulder that you wish to massage.
- Gently lean in towards the wall in order to apply some pressure from your roller into your muscles.
- Keeping upright, move your upper body gently forwards and backwards, left to right and right to left along your roller, so that you feel your muscles being pulled or nudged by the roller. The roller stays still.
- Maintain a steady, consistent pressure from the roller on to your muscles as you gently pull the muscle fibres side to side to loosen them.
- To do this massage around the front and back of your shoulder and upper arm, turn yourself either slightly away from or towards the wall.
- Work into any area for up to 30 seconds, focusing on areas that feel restricted, tight or knotted.
- Repeat on your right shoulder.
- Keep your shoulders down and relaxed. Start with a light roller pressure into your muscles and increase slowly for a deeper massage. Your roller should be nudging and moving your muscles a little, rather than pulling your skin, so lean in on the roller until you feel it in your muscles.

> You will feel pressure and a slight pulling sensation in the muscles directly under the roller and slightly to either side as you ease restrictions in the tissues. The area may feel warm as you work into it.

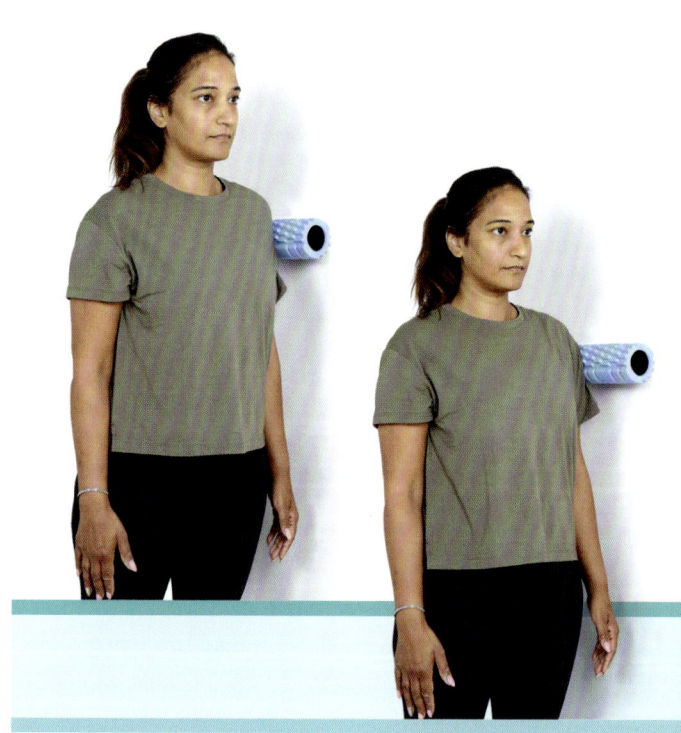

SHOULDER MOVEMENTS, STRETCHES AND SELF-MASSAGES

ⓡ Shoulder blade muscle massage

The rotator cuff is a group of muscles that get tight from desk work, computer use and driving. This massage loosens tight or knotted muscles and helps to keep or restore full and free movement, which in turn reduces strain on the joint.

- Stand in as good as neutral posture (*see* p. 35) as you can, with your left side to the wall and turning away from it slightly.
- Cup your left hand behind the back of your head to make the area to be massaged accessible.
- Place a massage roller between the wall and the back of the outer part of your left shoulder blade.
- Gently lean in towards the wall to apply some pressure from the roller into your muscles.
- Stay upright and lower yourself by bending and straightening your legs 3–10 times, to apply a rolling massage to the lower rotator cuff muscles, maintaining a steady, gentle pressure.
- To release stickiness between the layers of your muscles, you can also do a muscle-pulling, cross-fibre massage into the same area. Keep the roller still and move your upper body a short distance forwards and backwards, left and right and right and left along your roller 3–5 times.
- Repeat on the other side.
- **Start massaging gently, as this can often be a sensitive area, then slowly increase the pressure to gain a deeper massage. You can move the massage roller to different levels in this area of your body and repeat both types of massage.**

> Putting your hand behind your head gives the muscles a slight pre-stretch, so you may feel the effect as soon as you lean on to the roller. When rolling you will feel a pressure wave effect directly under the roller. When doing the cross-fibre massage you will feel pressure and a slight pulling sensation in the muscles directly under the roller and slightly to either side of it.

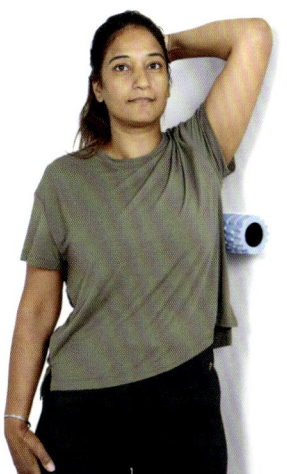
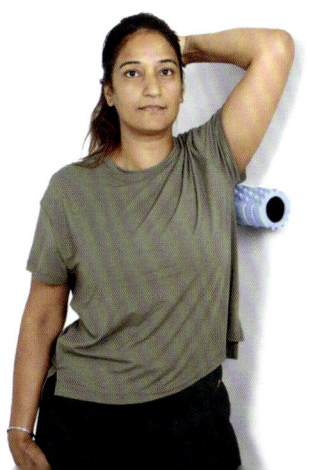
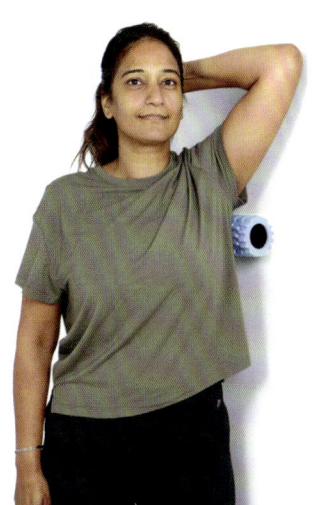
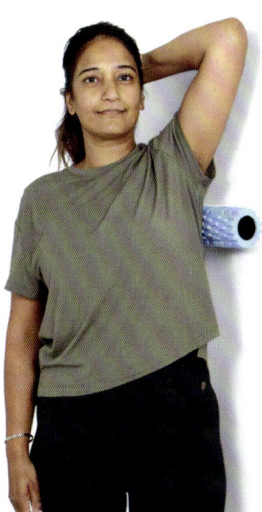

ⓡ Top of shoulder massage

This simple self-massage technique enables you to massage the top of your shoulders, loosening tight or knotted muscles and helping to restore full and free movement, which reduces strain on the joint. As well as a massage roller or pole, you'll need a resistance band or towel. By using a lever effect you can make this massage as deep or as light as you want.

- Sit tall in neutral posture (*see* p. 38) on a reasonably firm chair.
- Loop a resistance band around one end of a roller or, if you're using a pole, secure a towel around it, to create a massage texture.

You will feel the massage in your muscles on top of your shoulders and the lower part of the side and back of your neck. Once you get more familiar with the technique you can even use it to massage the very top of your upper back either side of your spine, which is a difficult-to-reach area.

- Sit with the ends of the band under your left buttock and place the roller on top of your right shoulder, with the band passing behind your back.
- Hold the front end of the roller with your left hand – the opposite one to the side being massaged – so that the shoulder being massaged can open and relax down.
- Change the position of the roller or tighten or loosen the band a little to adjust the pressure into your shoulder until you find what's right for you.
- Repeat on the other shoulder.
- **Try to relax your shoulders back and down and start with a light pressure. You can increase the intensity of the massage by tightening your band or positioning the roller to give a longer lever, but you don't need hard pressure for a massage that unsticks your muscles effectively. Make sure you don't massage directly on your bones.**

MORE SHOULDER SELF-MASSAGES

To ease areas that are painful, increase your freedom of movement in tight areas or improve blood flow you can also try the following shoulder self-massages, on their own or in combination:

UP AND DOWN MASSAGE

Find a tight knot or point on the top of your shoulder and position the massage roller directly on it. Pull the front end of the pole or roller down towards the floor to apply pressure. Hold for 5–10 seconds, release and then repeat. Then move the roller to a different tight area of your muscles and do it again. There will be a mildly achy, but not painful, pressure as you pull down and hold, followed by an easing as you release.

SHAKER MASSAGE

Create a loosening muscle massage at any point on the top of your shoulder by shaking your massage roller with small, fast, forwards-and-backwards movements into your muscle for up to 10 seconds. Move the roller to different positions to loosen other tight areas. You will feel pressure, a slightly warm sensation and your muscles being gently jiggled loose.

ROLLING PIN MASSAGE

Place your massage roller on your shoulder near your neck. Roll it out across the top of your shoulder, away from your neck and then back towards your neck. Do this repeatedly for up to 10 seconds. You will feel a gentle pressure just in front of and under the roller as it rolls across your upper shoulder area.

9 TARGETED EXERCISE COMBINATIONS

TARGETED EXERCISE COMBINATIONS

As we've explained, with the Make Movement Your Medicine method you can do any exercise on its own at any time and in any place, and it will make a positive difference to your body. However, we appreciate that some people prefer to have a little more direction, so in this chapter we have put together a range of carefully selected exercise combinations for you.

It is vital to maintain movement in the upper back, from the base of the neck to the base of the ribs, as otherwise neck and shoulder strains and upper back ache are much more likely. For this reason we have included exercises covering the three main upper back movements of flexion/extension, side bending and rotation in each of the combinations in this chapter.

We have organised the sequences into groups based on:

- How much time you have (*see* pp. 118–129)
- What your situation is and the areas of your body that really need to function well – or where you may be experiencing pain (*see* pp. 130–153)
- Common issues that you might want to focus on (*see* pp. 154–171)

When you combine our exercises into short sequences they become even more powerful. We have given you a choice of two options for each table of movements, stretches and self-massages. You don't have to do both sequences at once, but you could try them on different days to ring the changes or see which you prefer. Or you could do both, if you have time – the more, the better!

We want to encourage you to experiment, so think of these sequences as examples and as you learn what works for you and what you enjoy, use them as models for developing your own sequences. What's most important, though, is that you simply start!

For a full list of exercise combinations please see the directory on p. 175.

TOP TIP

After completing the tightness tests (*see* Chapter 5) you may find that you have restrictions in particular areas of your upper body. If you do the suggested exercises that follow and retest yourself, you will be able to note your improvement. This can help to motivate you and assess exactly which movements work best for you.

ESSENTIAL WARM-UP EXERCISES

If you only have a few minutes – perhaps you're taking a very quick work break or waiting for the kettle to boil – the best thing you can do to help yourself is to reduce your upper back/spine stiffness with the essential warm-up exercises in table 9.1. This is because upper back stiffness is very often the root cause of neck and shoulder pain as well as upper back discomfort. If you do nothing else but these three exercises daily, then you will be doing yourself a big favour: they really can change how you feel and function throughout your life.

These exercises should also be done before you do any of the other sequences, just to ensure your body is properly prepared.

Table 9.1 Essential warm-up exercises

Exercise name	Page
Upper back easer A or Upper back round and lift	60 or 66
Upper back rotation, seated or Upper back rotation, standing	62 or 61
Rib opener stretch	70

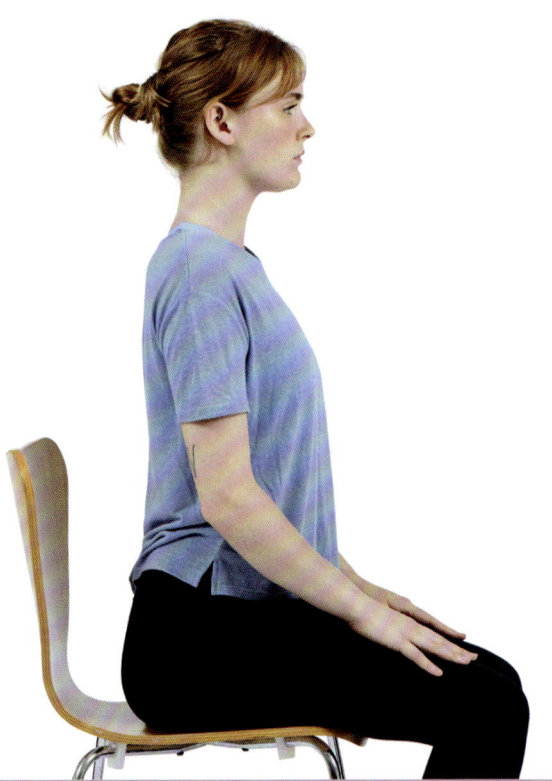

Upper back easer A or Upper back round and lift

TARGETED EXERCISE COMBINATIONS

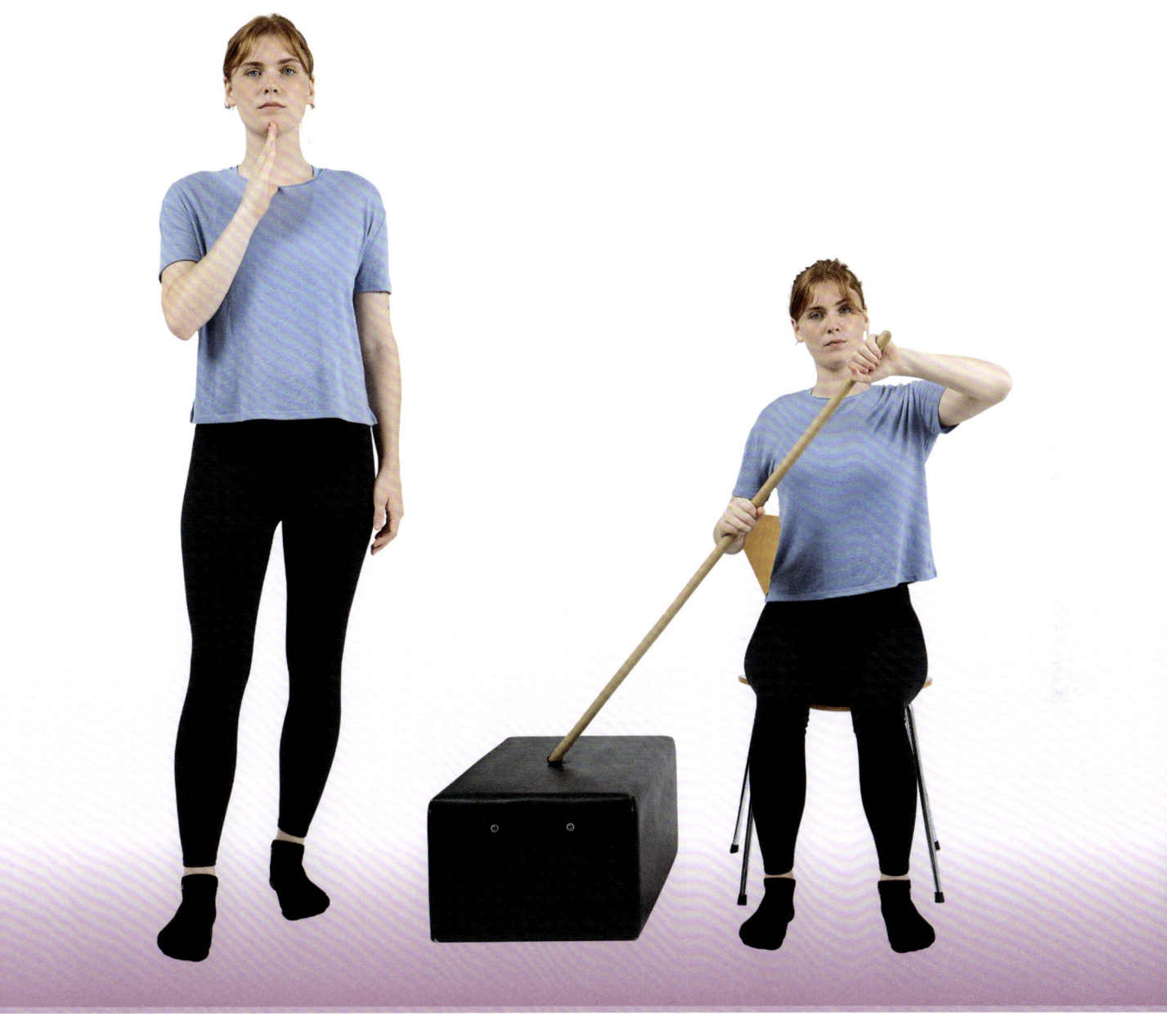

Upper back rotation, standing or Upper back rotation, seated

Rib opener stretch

MAKE MOVEMENT YOUR MEDICINE

QUICK SEQUENCES

If you've got a little longer to help yourself, try adding one of the sequences from tables 9.2, 9.3 or 9.4 that follow, as well as doing the warm-up exercises in table 9.1. These include additional targeted exercises for your upper back, neck or shoulders, depending on the area you would like help for. What's great is that you can repeat these quick routines several times a day.

Upper back

Doing these sequences will reduce pain from sitting or slouching for long periods. Releasing muscle tension and improving posture will make your back feel lighter, more comfortable, more mobile and healthier.

Choose one of the following options (or try both!) after doing the essential warm-up movements in table 9.1 (*see* p. 116):

Table 9.2

Option 1	Page
Chest lift	65
Two-arm forward hang, seated	71
Rib shifter	59
Spinal muscle massage	74
Option 2	**Page**
Two-arm swipe	67
Chest and shoulder release A or B	72 or 73
Upper back easer A	60
Side of back massage	76

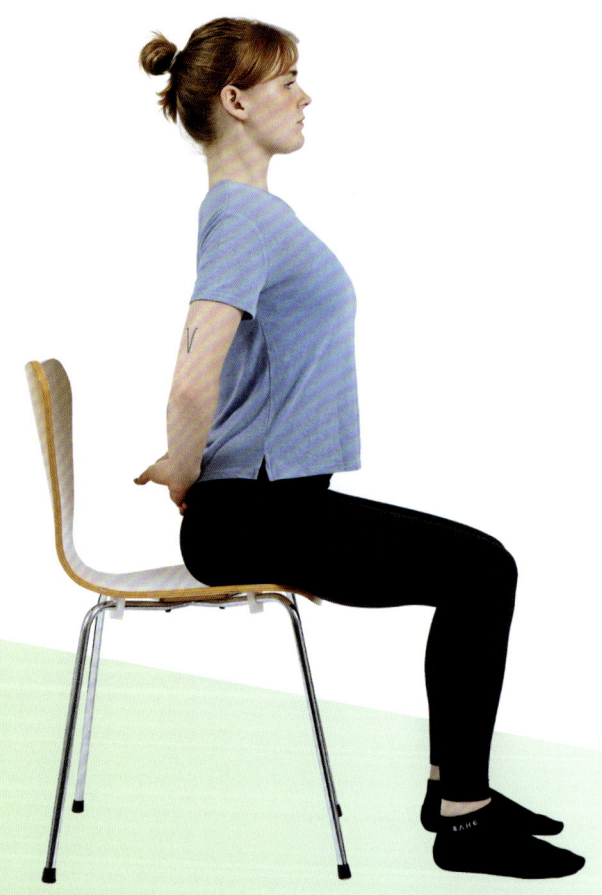

TARGETED EXERCISE COMBINATIONS

Upper back option 1

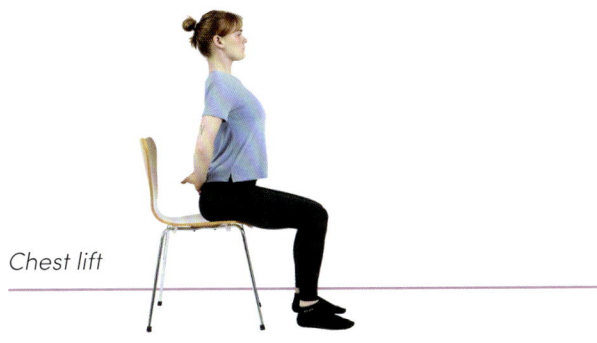

Chest lift

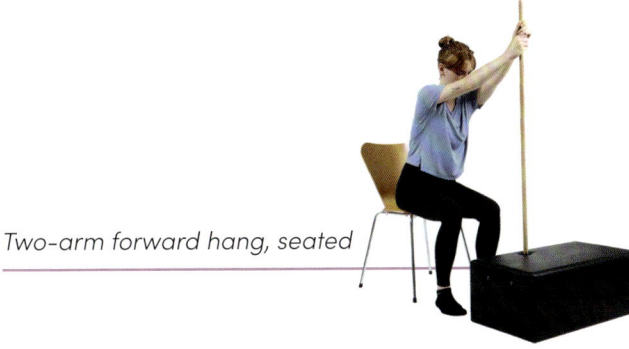

Two-arm forward hang, seated

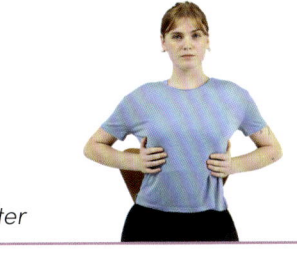

Rib shifter

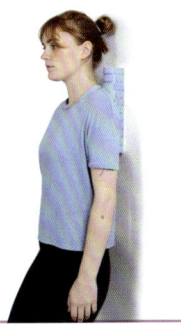

Spinal muscle massage

Upper back option 2

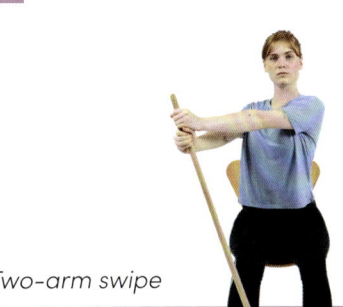

Two-arm swipe

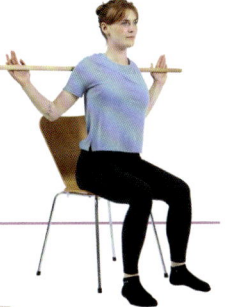

Chest and shoulder release A or B

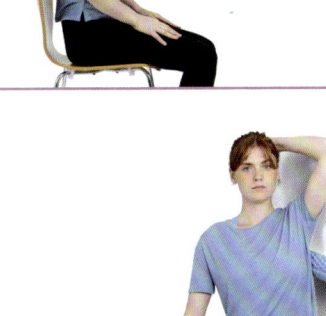

Upper back easer A

Side of back massage

119

Neck

These sequences help to relieve stress and stiffness in your neck from overworked muscles. They help to correct poor posture and to maintain good long-term head and neck alignment. Regular practice can prevent muscle tension and restore mobility, particularly for those who use tech or round forward for their work or hobbies.

Choose one of the following options (or try both!) after doing the essential warm-up movements in table 9.1 (*see* p. 116):

Table 9.3

Option 1	Page
Slide the chin in	83
Back of neck stretch A	85
Neck settling movements × 3	81
Nodding neck massage	90
Option 2	**Page**
Neck saucer glide	84
Decompress your neck	88
Neck settling movements × 3	81
Rotating neck massage	91

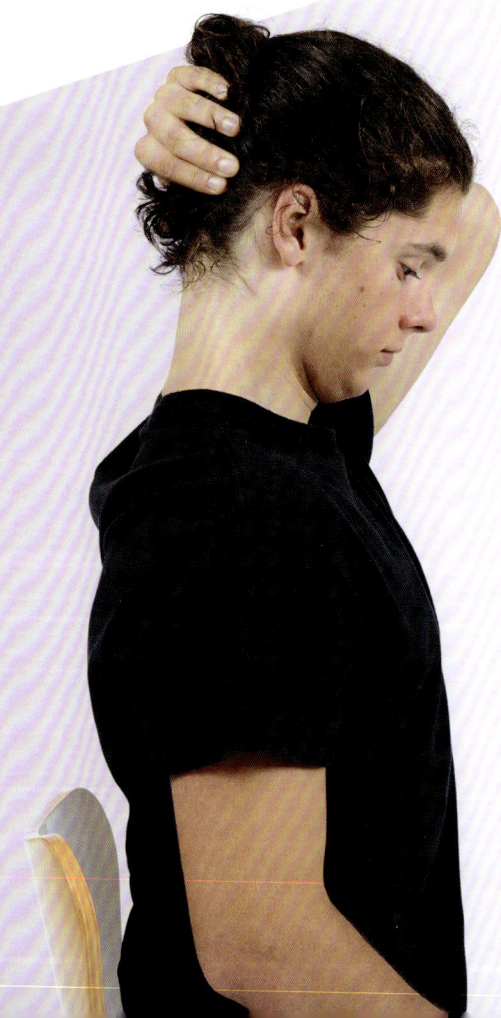

TARGETED EXERCISE COMBINATIONS

Neck option 1

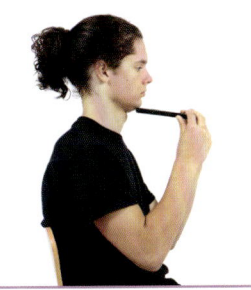
Slide the chin in

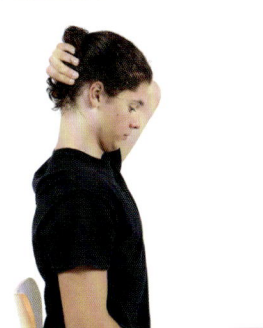
Back of neck stretch A

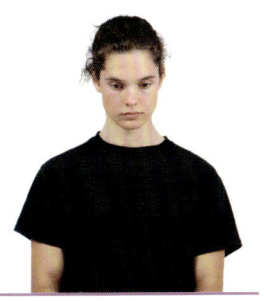
Neck settling movements × 3

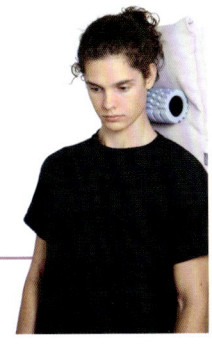
Nodding neck massage

Neck option 2

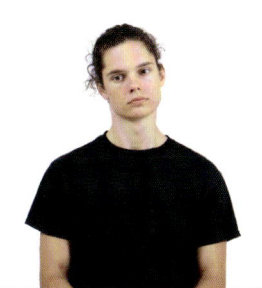
Neck saucer glide

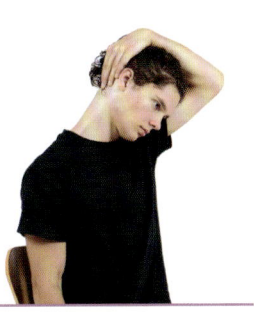
Decompress your neck

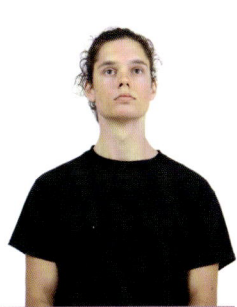
Neck settling movements × 3

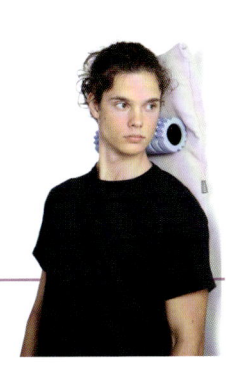
Rotating neck massage

Shoulders

These sequences can help your shoulders by relieving pain and easing tension caused by repetitive use, poor positioning or chronic tightness. They will help to restore mobility and good posture by easing tightness in the muscles and joints. By regularly doing the sequences you will increase range of motion and comfort.

Choose one of the following options (or try both!) after doing the essential warm-up movements in table 9.1 (*see* p. 116):

Table 9.4

Option 1	Page
Shoulder blade squeezer	103
One-arm forward hang, standing or seated	104
Horizontal arm circles	96
Shoulder rolling massage	109
Option 2	**Page**
Cross-body reach	100
Back scratcher	108
Push forward, pull back	97
Shoulder blade muscle massage	111

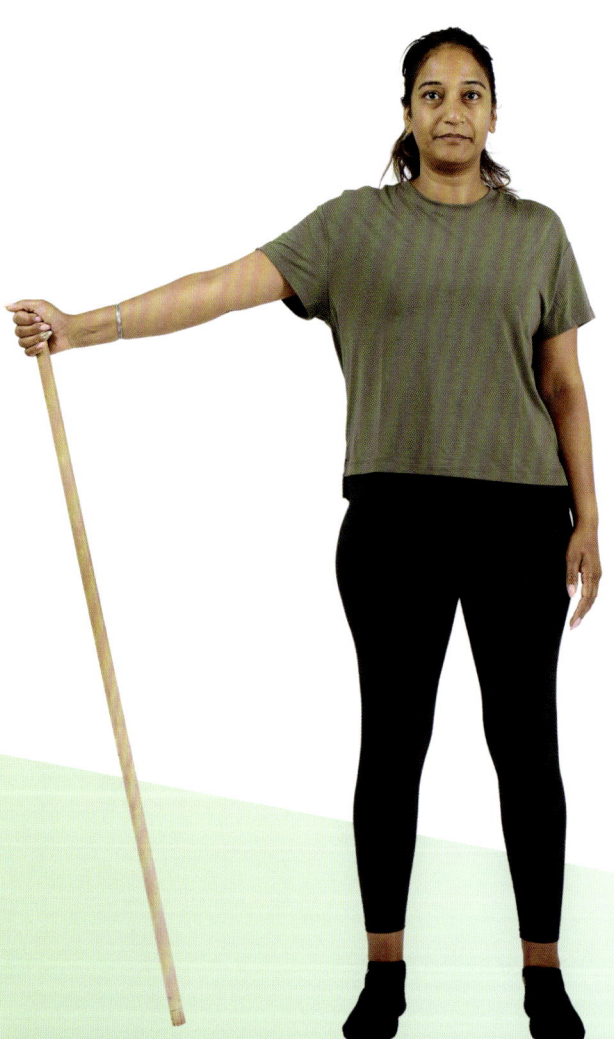

TARGETED EXERCISE COMBINATIONS

Shoulder option 1

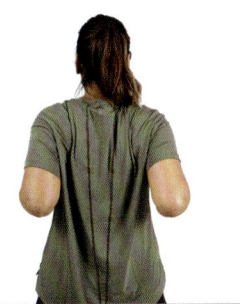

Shoulder blade squeezer

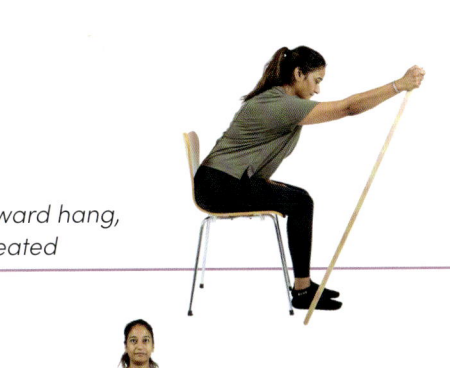

One-arm forward hang, standing or seated

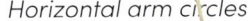

Horizontal arm circles

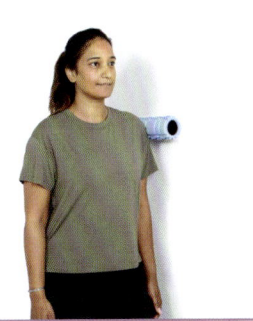

Shoulder rolling massage

Shoulder option 2

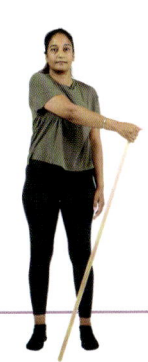

Cross-body reach

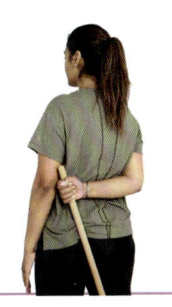

Back scratcher

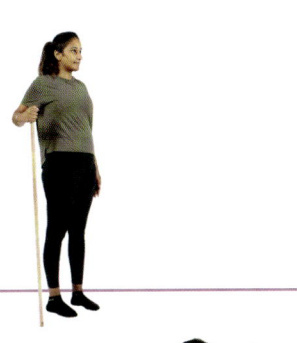

Push forward, pull back

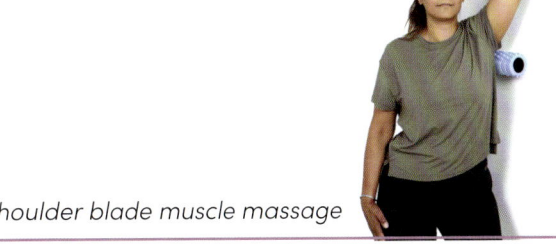

Shoulder blade muscle massage

LONGER SEQUENCES

Tables 9.5, 9.6 and 9.7 provide some longer sequences for those with a bit more time to devote to movement medicine. As before, start with the essential warm-up movements, then choose one of the options below, according to your target area.

Upper back

As keeping the upper back functioning well is so important, if you have some additional time you could try one of the sequences below. This will help to restore good posture and make your upper back, neck and shoulders more comfortable.

Choose one of the following options (or try both!) after doing the essential warm-up movements in table 9.1 (*see* p. 116):

Table 9.5

Option 1	Page
Rib release	64
Desk chest stretch	69
Rib shifter	59
Spinal muscle massage	74
Upper back easer B	68
Option 2	**Page**
Upper back rotation, lying	63
Rib opener stretch	70
Upper back easer A	60
Side of back massage	76
Two-arm swipe	67

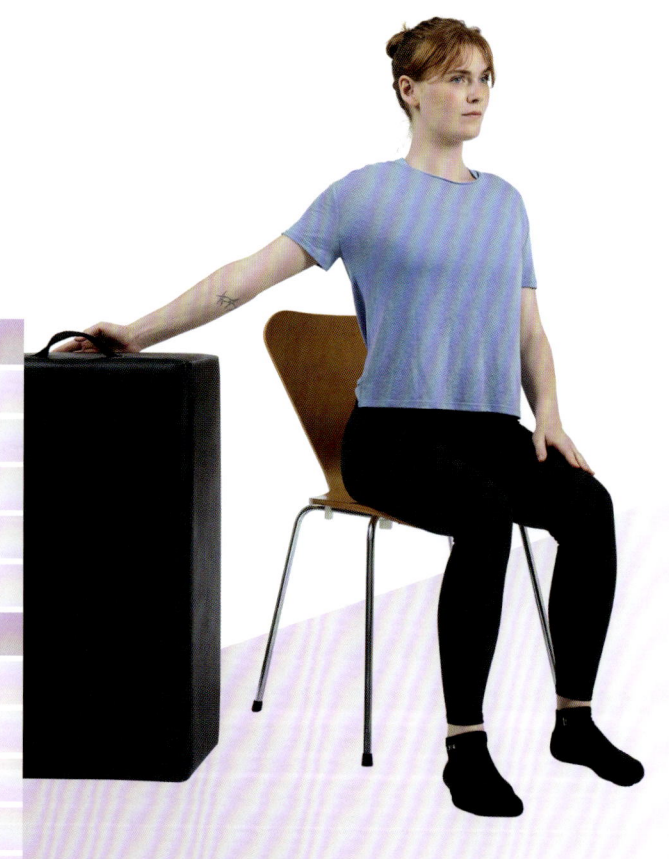

TARGETED EXERCISE COMBINATIONS

Upper back option 1

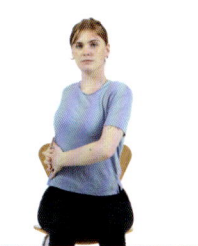
Rib release

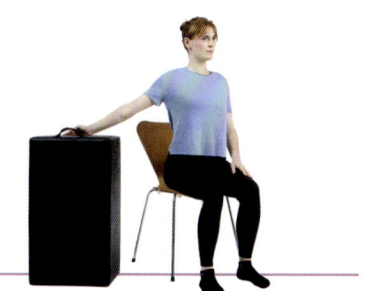
Desk chest stretch

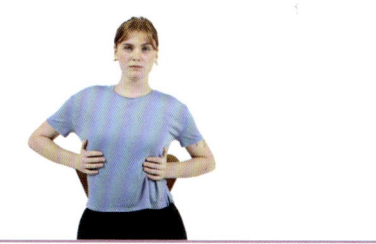
Rib shifter

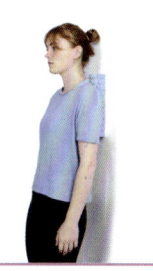
Spinal muscle massage

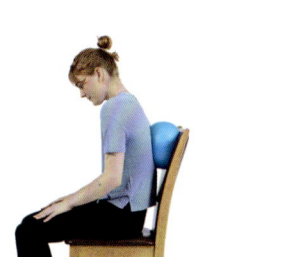
Upper back easer B

Upper back option 2

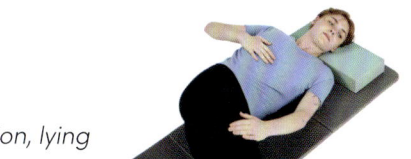
Upper back rotation, lying

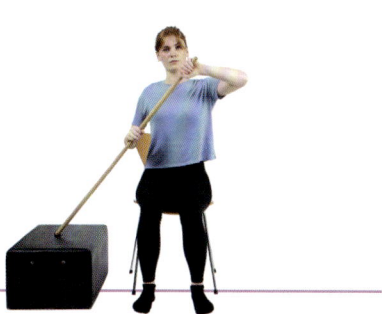
Rib opener stretch

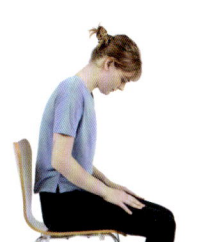
Upper back easer A

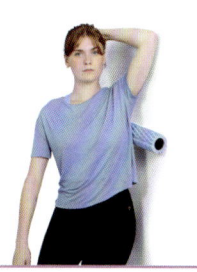
Side of back massage

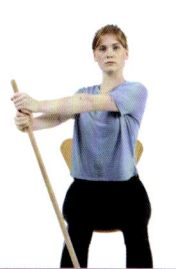
Two-arm swipe

125

Neck

As with the shorter sequences, the longer sequences below will also help to relieve stress and stiffness in your neck. They help to correct poor posture and to maintain good long-term head and neck alignment. Regular practice can prevent muscle tension and restore mobility, particularly for those who use tech or round forward for their work or hobbies.

Choose one of the following options (or try both!) after doing the essential warm-up movements in table 9.1 (*see* p. 116):

Table 9.6

Option 1	Page
Turn right, turn left	82
De-stress your neck	87
Neck settling movements × 3	81
Lying down neck massage	92
Neck saucer glide	84
Option 2	**Page**
Slide the chin in	83
Release your neck	89
Neck settling movements × 3	81
Nodding neck massage	90
Neck saucer glide	84

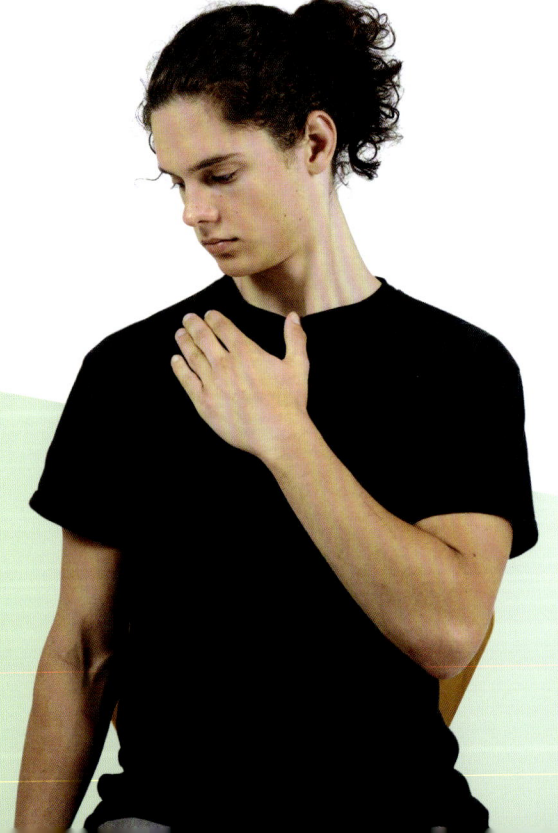

TARGETED EXERCISE COMBINATIONS

Neck option 1

Turn right, turn left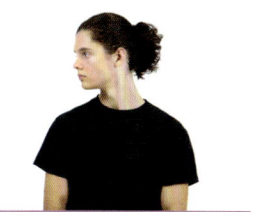

De-stress your neck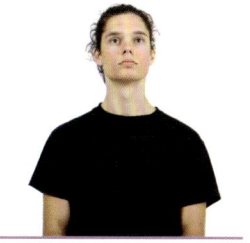

Neck settling movements × 3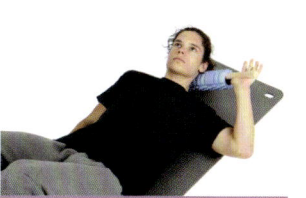

Lying down neck massage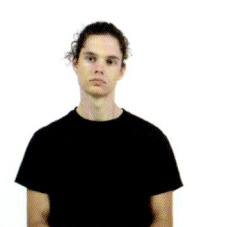

Neck saucer glide

Neck option 2

Slide the chin in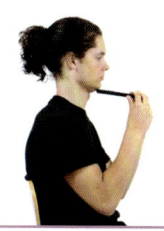

Release your neck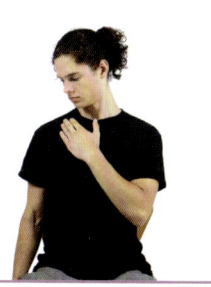

Neck settling movements × 3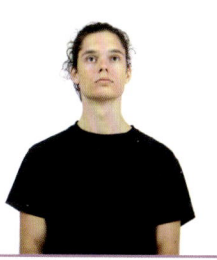

Nodding neck massage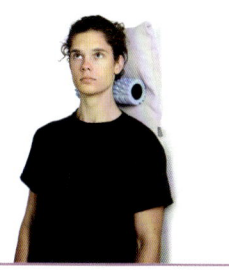

Neck saucer glide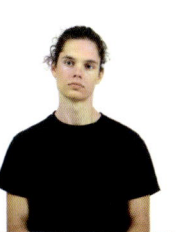

MAKE MOVEMENT YOUR MEDICINE

Shoulders

As with the shorter sequences, these slightly longer sequences can help your shoulders by relieving pain and easing tension caused by repetitive use, poor positioning or chronic tightness. They will help to restore mobility and good posture by easing tightness in the muscles and joints. By regularly doing the sequences you will increase range of motion and comfort.

Choose one of the following options (or try both!) after doing the essential warm-up movements in table 9.1 (*see* p. 116):

Table 9.7

Option 1	Page
Underarm swing	102
Side hang, standing or seated	106
Push forward, pull back	97
Shoulder cross-fibre massage	110
Pendulum swing front	98
Option 2	**Page**
Put your coat on	101
Across-body hang, standing or seated	105
Horizontal arm circles	96
Top of shoulder massage	112
Pendulum swing behind	99

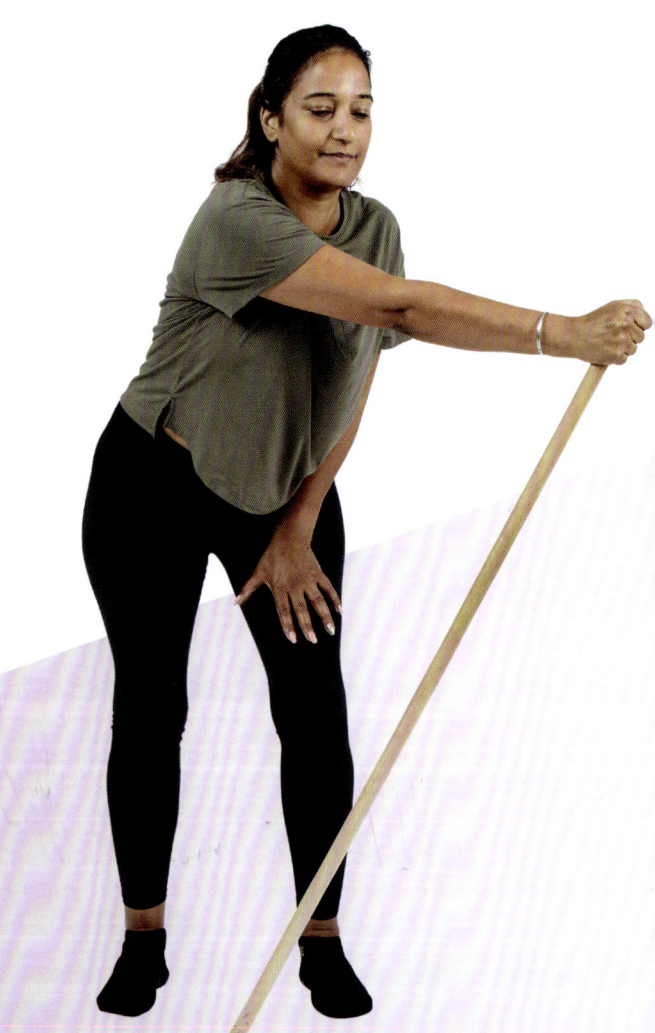

TARGETED EXERCISE COMBINATIONS

Shoulders option 1

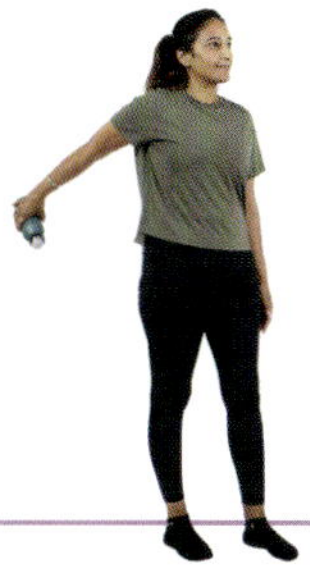

Underarm swing

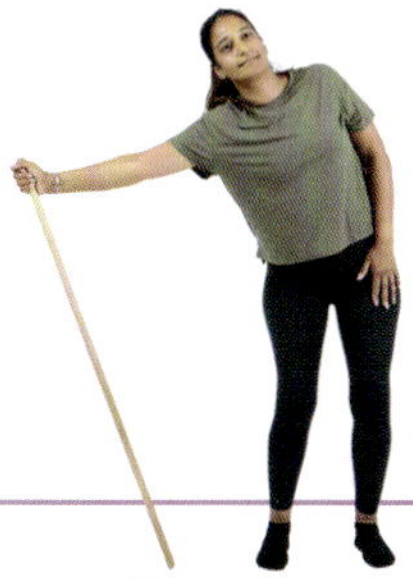

Side hang, standing or seated

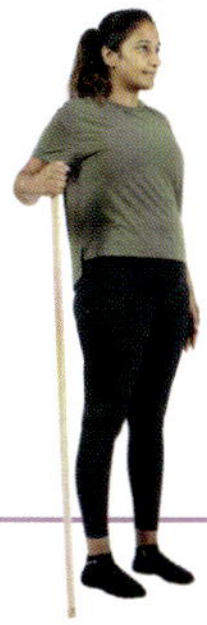

Push forward, pull back

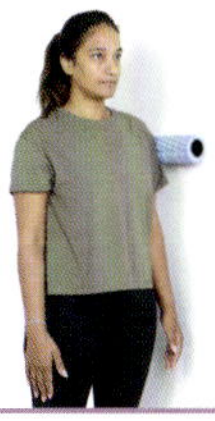

Shoulder cross-fibre massage

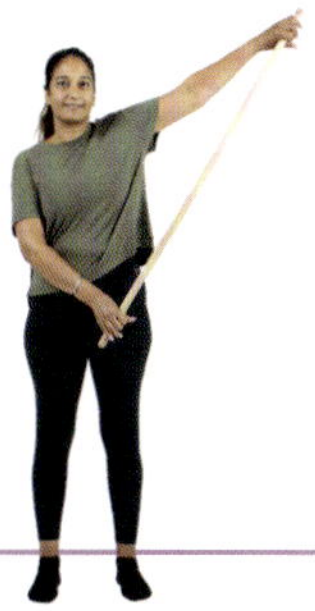

Pendulum swing front

Shoulders option 2

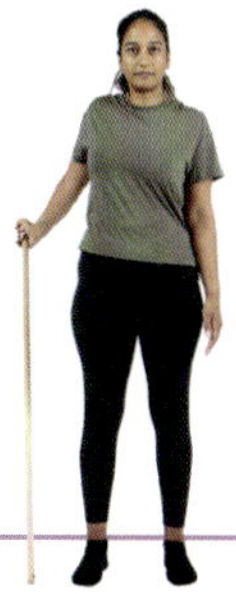

Put your coat on

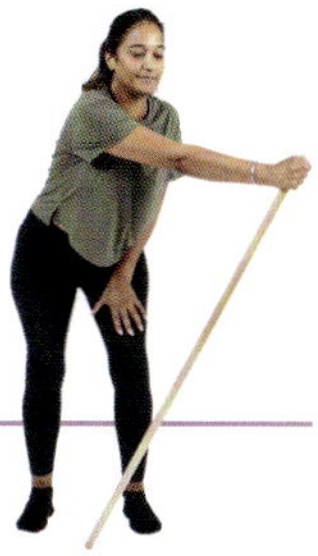

Across-body hang, standing or seated

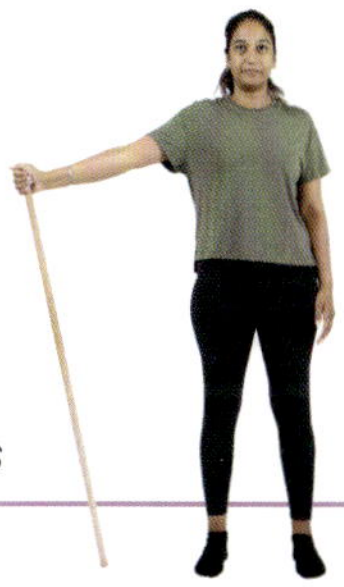

Horizontal arm circles

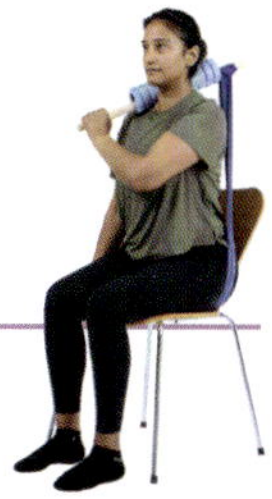

Top of shoulder massage

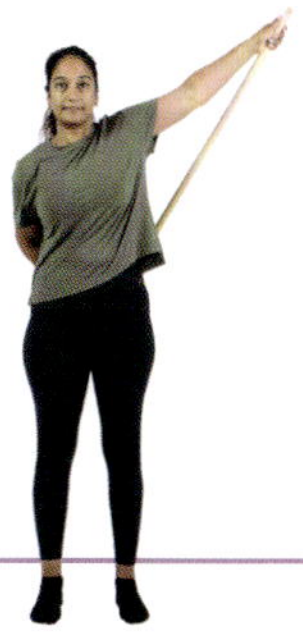

Pendulum swing behind

SEQUENCES FOR DIFFERENT SCENARIOS

In this section, you'll find exercises for all sorts of scenarios that can cause issues in the upper back, neck and shoulders. We've arranged them by whether they relate to work, lifestyle, hobbies or sports. Although we can't cover everything, we've tried to include a broad range of common situations so that you can find a sequence that suits you.

Whoever you are and whatever situation you find yourself in, we want to remind you to start small, stay consistent and be aware of how your body feels. If you want to retain mobility and avoid pain in your upper body it is essential to move, and each movement, stretch or massage will help you live a healthier and happier life.

For the office worker

If you're an office worker you probably end up sitting in one position for hours, and poor posture and repetitive movements can result in neck pain, especially if you're stiff in your upper back. These exercise combinations only take a few minutes to do, but they can help head off pain and if you're in extreme discomfort they may give you immediate relief. If the pain is very strong, apply a heat or cold pack, as you prefer, to your neck to soothe your muscles *(see active pain relief, p. 25)* and repeat one of the options every 30 to 60 minutes.

Choose one of the following options (or try both!) after doing the essential warm-up movements in table 9.1 *(see p. 116)*:

Table 9.8

Option 1	Page
Neck saucer glide	84
Back of neck stretch A	85
Neck settling movements × 3	81
Rotating neck massage	91
Two-arm forward hang, seated	71
Upper back easer A	60
Option 2	**Page**
Turn right, turn left	82
Decompress your neck	88
Neck settling movements × 3	81
Rib release	64
Release your neck	89
Neck settling movements × 3	81

TARGETED EXERCISE COMBINATIONS

For the office worker option 1

Neck saucer glide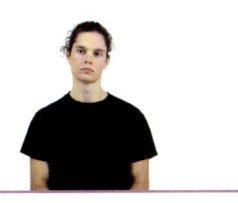

Back of neck stretch A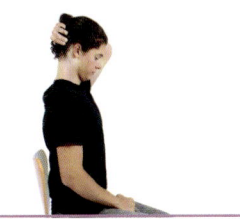

Neck settling movements × 3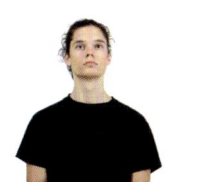

Rotating neck massage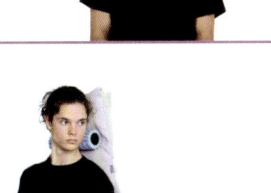

Two-arm forward hang, seated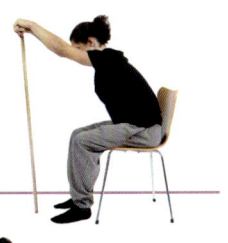

Upper back easer A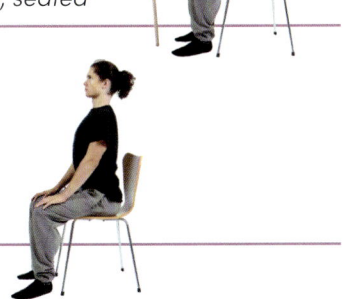

For the office worker option 2

Turn right, turn left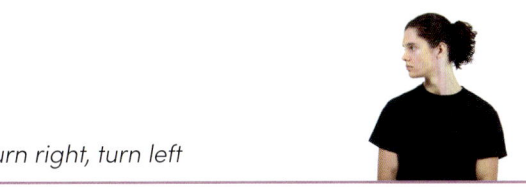

Decompress your neck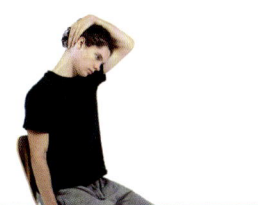

Neck settling movements × 3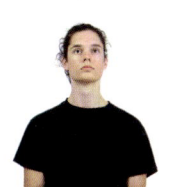

Rib release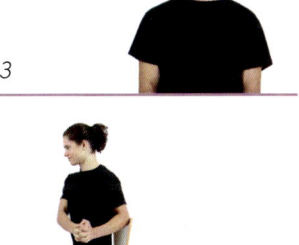

Release your neck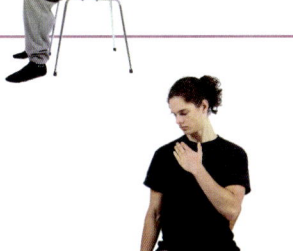

Neck settling movements × 3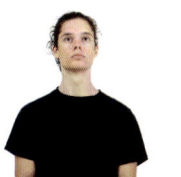

MAKE MOVEMENT YOUR MEDICINE

For someone standing on their feet all day

If you are required to stand for much of the day it is likely that your posture will suffer. This can lead to upper back, neck and shoulder strains.

To restore healthy movement to your upper body, choose one of the following options (or try both!) after doing the essential warm-up movements in table 9.1 (*see* p. 116):

Table 9.9

Option 1	Page
Shoulder blade squeezer	103
Across-body hang, standing or seated	105
Horizontal arm circles	96
Shoulder blade muscle massage	111
Rib opener stretch	70
Rib shifter	59
Option 2	**Page**
Put your coat on	101
Backward hang	107
Push forward, pull back	97
Top of shoulder massage	112
Release your neck	89
Neck settling movements × 3	81

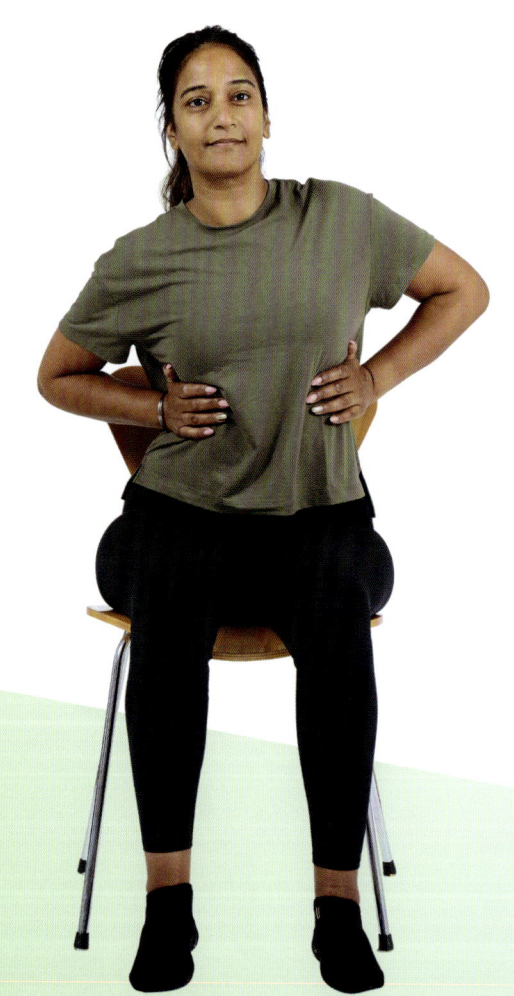

TARGETED EXERCISE COMBINATIONS

For someone standing on their feet all day option 1

Shoulder blade squeezer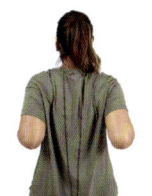

Across-body hang, standing or seated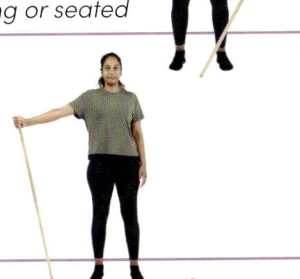

Horizontal arm circles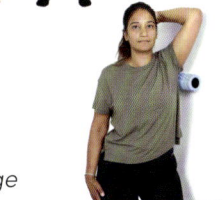

Shoulder blade muscle massage

Rib opener stretch

Rib shifter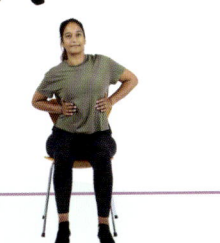

For someone standing on their feet all day option 2

Put your coat on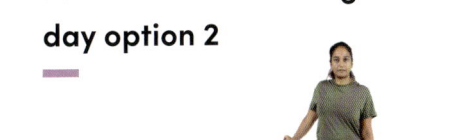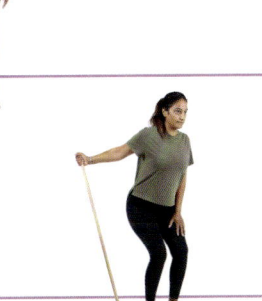

Backward hang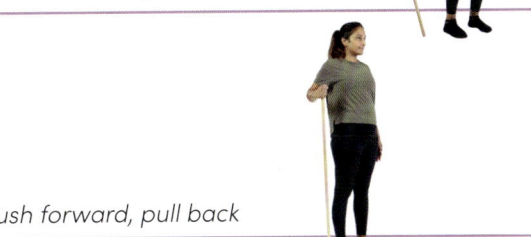

Push forward, pull back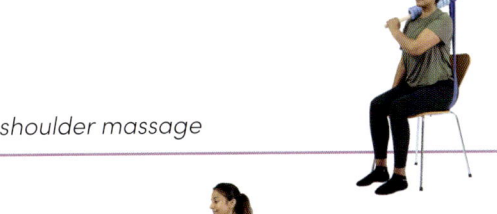

Top of shoulder massage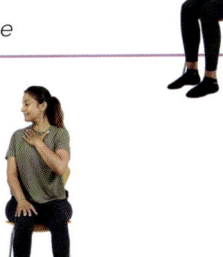

Release your neck

Neck settling movements × 3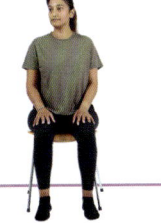

133

For tradespeople and DIYers

People working in the trades, such as carpenters, plumbers, electricians and builders, together with DIYers at home, put a lot of physical demands on their upper bodies. The often awkward positions they are forced to work in, together with twisting and lifting, can cause muscle imbalances, aches and pains.

To counteract these, choose one of the following options (or try both!) after doing the essential warm-up movements in table 9.1 (*see* p. 116):

Table 9.10

Option 1	Page
Rib release	64
Across-body hang, standing or seated	105
Horizontal arm circles	96
Shoulder blade muscle massage	111
Two-arm forward hang, seated	71
Rib shifter	59
Option 2	**Page**
Chest lift	65
Decompress your neck	88
Neck settling movements × 3	81
Side of back massage	76
Backward hang	107
Push forward, pull back	97

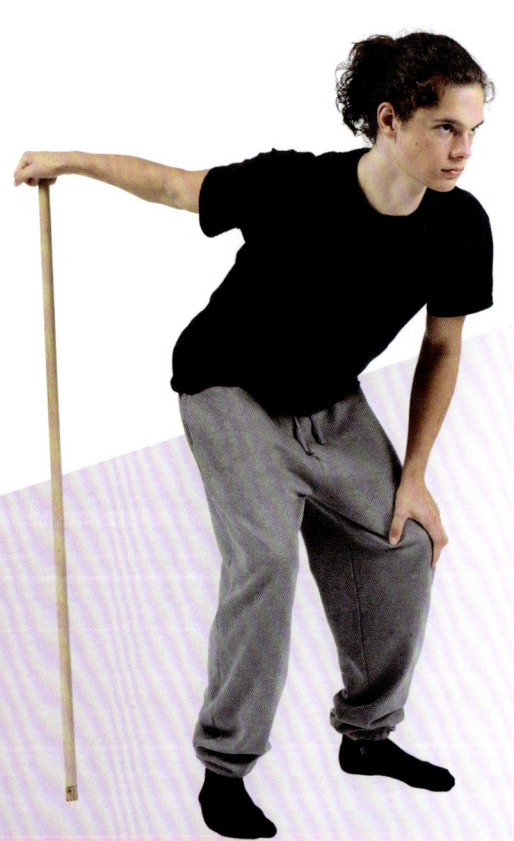

TARGETED EXERCISE COMBINATIONS

For tradespeople and DIYers option 1

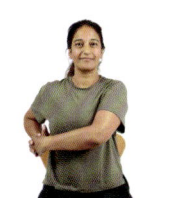
Rib release

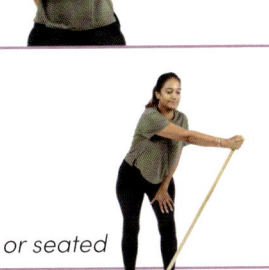
Across-body hang, standing or seated

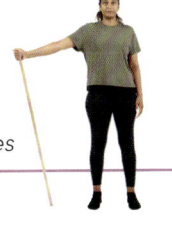
Horizontal arm circles

Shoulder blade muscle massage

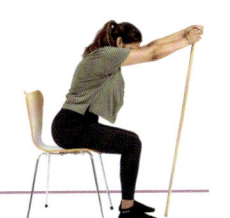
Two-arm forward hang, seated

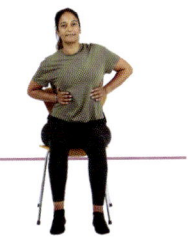
Rib shifter

For tradespeople and DIYersday option 2

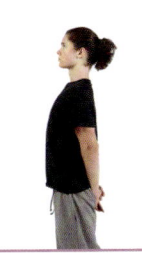
Chest lift

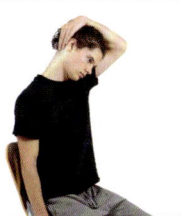
Decompress your neck

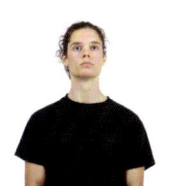
Neck settling movements × 3

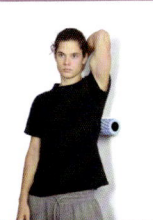
Side of back massage

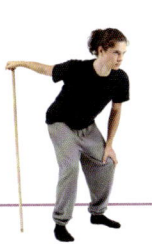
Backward hang

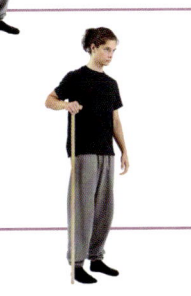
Push forward, pull back

MAKE MOVEMENT YOUR MEDICINE

For musicians and singers

The requirement to often hold an instrument or music score for long periods places extra demands on the upper back, neck and shoulders. Try the following combinations to prevent the build-up of tightness in your upper body when rehearsing and performing.

Choose one of the following options (or try both!) after doing the essential warm-up movements in table 9.1 (*see* p. 116):

Table 9.11

Option 1	Page
Shoulder blade squeezer	103
Release your neck	89
Neck settling movements × 3	81
Spinal muscle massage	74
Back scratcher	108
Horizontal arm circles	96

Option 2	Page
Turn right, turn left	82
Chest and shoulder release A or B	72 or 73
Upper back easer A or B	60 or 68
Top of shoulder massage	112
One-arm forward hang, standing or seated	104
Push forward, pull back	97

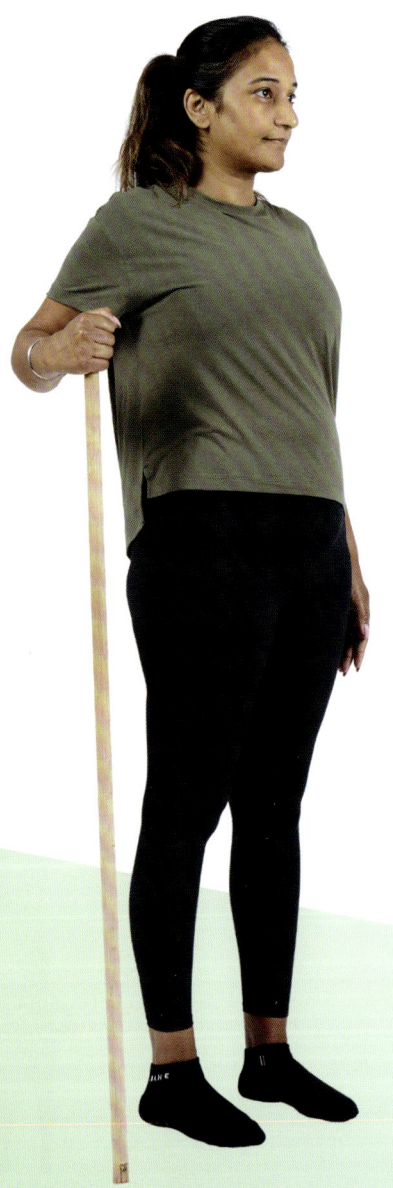

TARGETED EXERCISE COMBINATIONS

For musicians and singers option 1

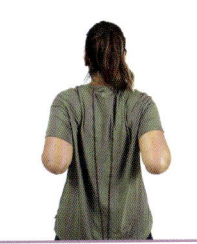
Shoulder blade squeezer

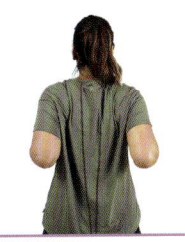
Release your neck

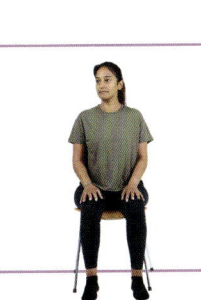
Neck settling movements x 3

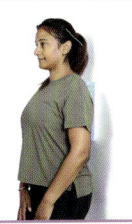
Spinal muscle massage

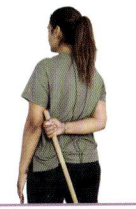
Back scratcher

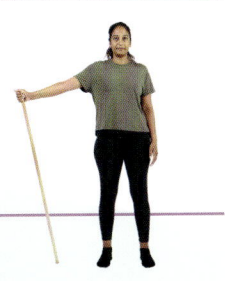
Horizontal arm circles

For musicians and singers option 2

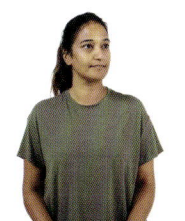
Turn right, turn left

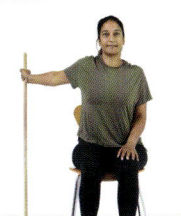
Chest and shoulder release A or B

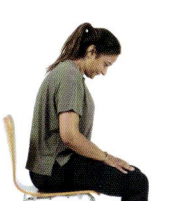
Upper back easer A or B

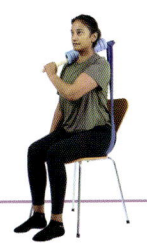
Top of shoulder massage

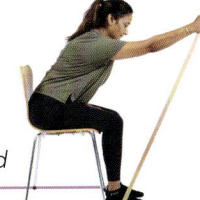
One-arm forward hang, standing or seated

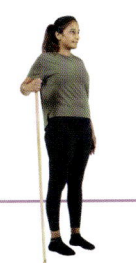
Push forward, pull back

MAKE MOVEMENT YOUR MEDICINE

For the new parent or grandparent

Caring for a baby puts new demands on your upper back, neck and shoulders, because you're carrying, bending, twisting and stretching in new ways. It's quite normal to experience some aches and pains while your body gets used to caring for the new infant. These exercise combinations will keep you mobile and, if you find you're in pain, help your pain melt away.

Choose one of the following options (or try both!) after doing the essential warm-up movements in table 9.1 (*see* p. 116):

Table 9.12

Option 1	Page
Chest lift	65
Chest and shoulder release A or B	72 or 73
Rib shifter	59
Shoulder rolling massage	109
Side hang, standing or seated	106
Horizontal arm circles	96
Option 2	**Page**
Shoulder blade squeezer	103
De-stress your neck	87
Neck settling movements × 3	81
Upper back massage	75
One-arm forward hang, standing or seated	104
Push forward, pull back	97

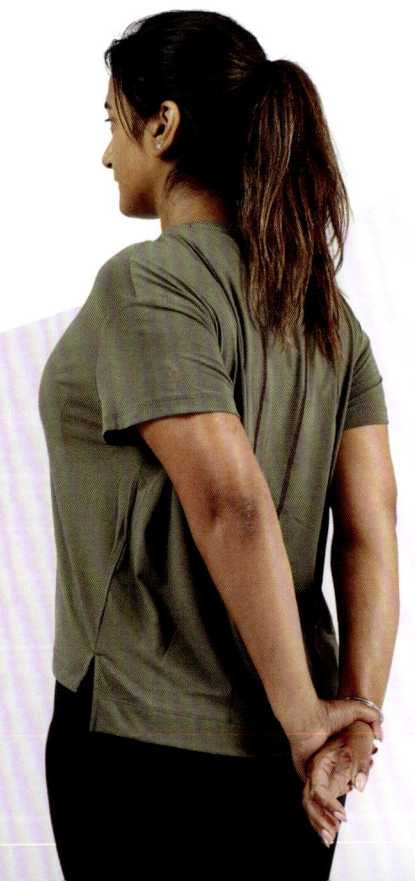

TARGETED EXERCISE COMBINATIONS

For the new parent or grandparent option 1

Chest lift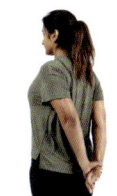

Chest and shoulder release A or B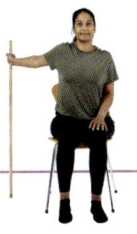

Rib shifter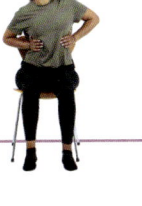

Shoulder rolling massage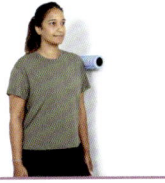

Side hang, standing or seated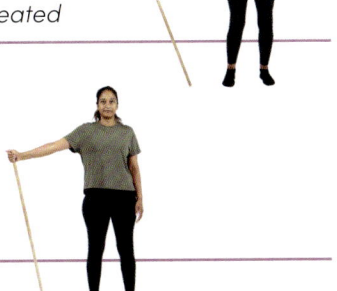

Horizontal arm circles

For the new parent or grandparent option 2

Shoulder blade squeezer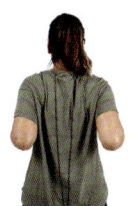

De-stress your neck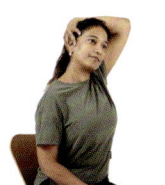

Neck settling movements × 3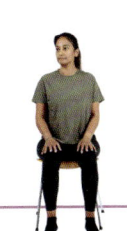

Upper back massage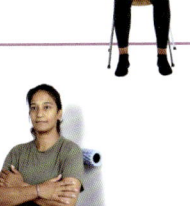

One-arm forward hang, standing or seated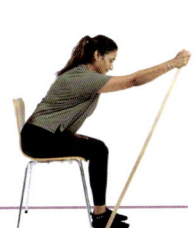

Push forward, pull back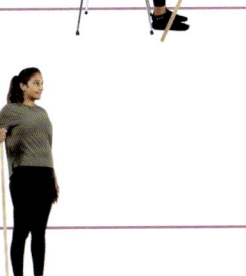

For the traveller

When you travel long distances, or even short ones, and you're unable to move as much as you should, your body can become stiff and ache. If you're in a car you can move when you stop for a break – for the desk chest stretch (see p. 69) you can use the car door frame to support you. In a train or plane the best way to keep your body comfortable is to move about every hour if possible. Of course, it's tricky if you're confined to your seat, but most of the exercise combinations can be done while sitting down. Try to utilise the space between carriages on a train or near the restroom area on a plane, although you will probably have to improvise without equipment like a pole. We have not included a massage in these combinations, as it may not be possible when travelling.

Choose one of the following options (or try both!) after doing the essential warm-up movements in table 9.1 (see p. 116):

Table 9.13

Option 1	Page
Turn right, turn left	82
Back of neck stretch A	85
Neck settling movements × 3	81
Chest lift	65
Desk chest stretch	69
Upper back easer A	60
Option 2	**Page**
Rib release	64
Back scratcher	108
Horizontal arm circles	96
Neck saucer glide	84
De-stress your neck	87
Neck settling movements × 3	81

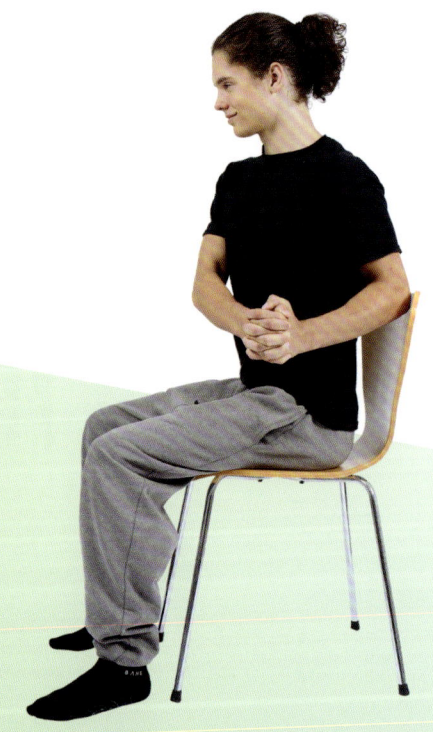

TARGETED EXERCISE COMBINATIONS

For the traveller option 1

Turn right, turn left

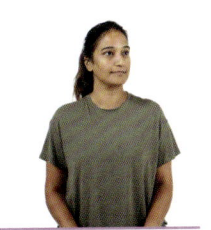

Back of neck stretch A

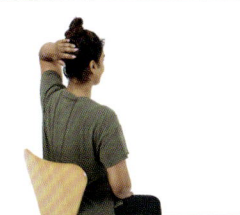

Neck settling movements × 3

Chest lift

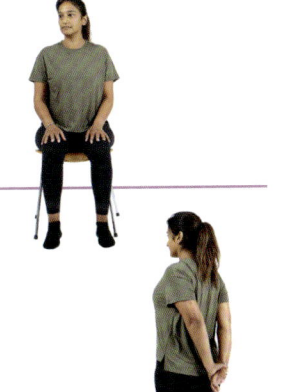

Desk chest stretch

Upper back easer A

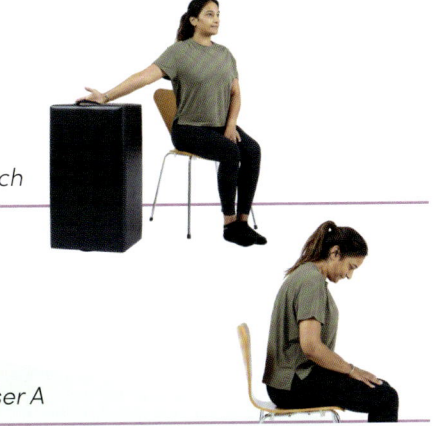

For the traveller option 2

Rib release

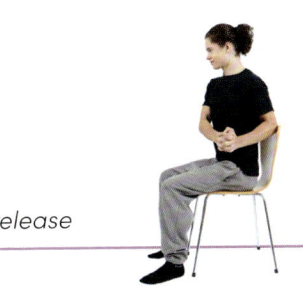

Back scratcher

Horizontal arm circles

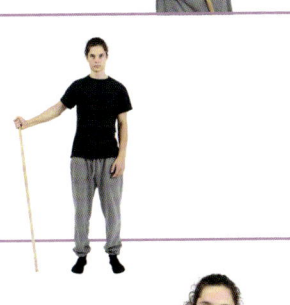

Neck saucer glide

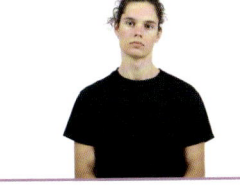

De-stress your neck

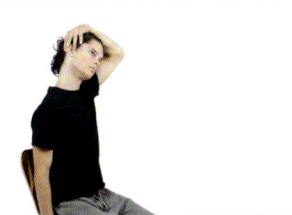

Neck settling movements × 3

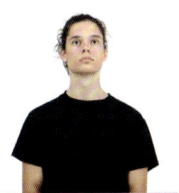

141

For the gamer

Even with a well-designed chair, gamers can spend a long time with rounded upper backs and shoulders, and their heads pushed forwards and their shoulders and backs rounded, particularly as the action gets intense! This can result in stiffness and pain in the upper body, so make sure you keep your ears over your shoulders as you game, as this will reduce neck strain. Take movement breaks as often as you can to run through a few movements, stretches and self-massages.

Choose one of the following options (or try both!) after doing the essential warm-up movements in table 9.1 (*see* p. 116):

Table 9.14

Option 1	Page
Slide the chin in	83
Release your neck	89
Neck settling movements × 3	81
Shoulder cross-fibre massage	110
Across-body hang, standing or seated	105
Horizontal arm circles	96
Option 2	**Page**
Put your coat on	101
Backward hang	107
Underarm swing	102
Spinal muscle massage	74
Decompress your neck	88
Neck settling movements × 3	81

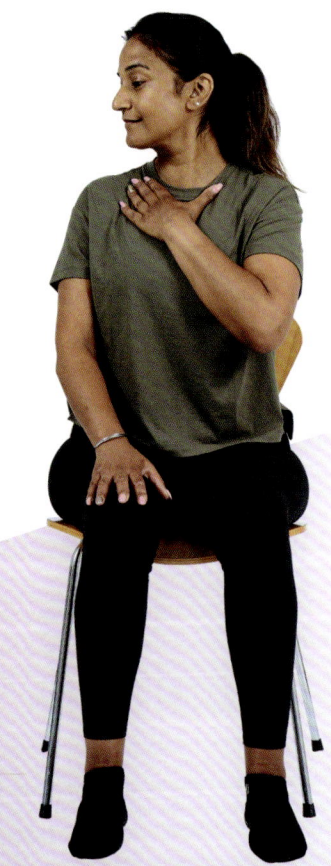

TARGETED EXERCISE COMBINATIONS

For the gamer option 1

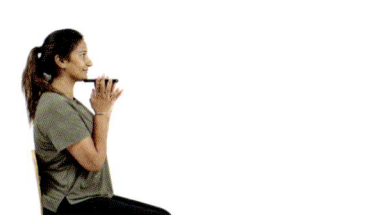
Slide the chin in

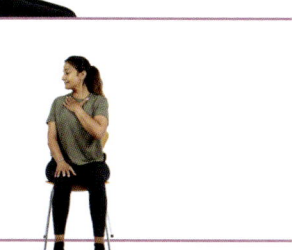
Release your neck

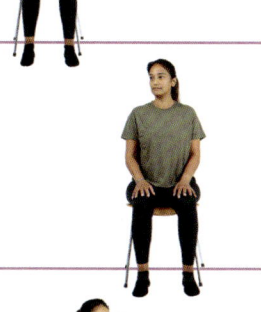
Neck settling movements × 3

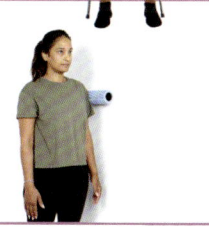
Shoulder cross-fibre massage

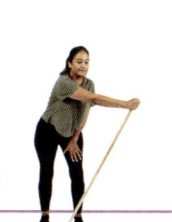
Across-body hang, standing or seated

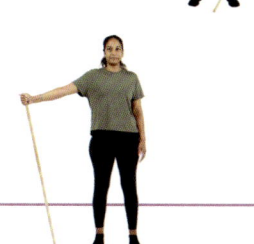
Horizontal arm circles

For the gamer option 2

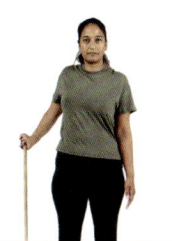
Put your coat on

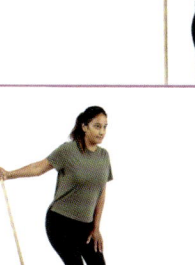
Backward hang

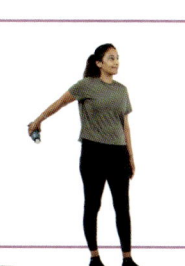
Underarm swing

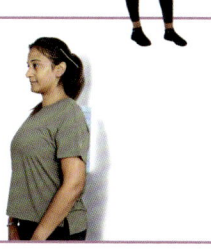
Spinal muscle massage

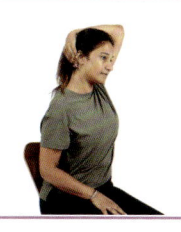
Decompress your neck

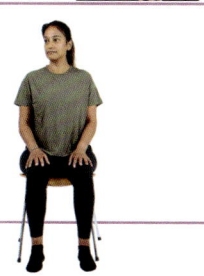
Neck settling movements × 3

For the gardener

It's easy to get carried away and garden for too long, often in a forward hunched posture, so it's beneficial to stop each hour and do some exercises. The following combinations will help restore your comfort, balance and good posture. By spending just a few minutes every hour doing this you will be able to get more done in the garden without becoming stiff and achy.

Choose one of the following options (or try both!) after doing the essential warm-up movements in table 9.1 (see p. 116):

Table 9.15

Option 1	Page
Chest lift	65
Chest and shoulder release A or B	72 or 73
Horizontal arm circles	96
Upper back massage	75
One-arm forward hang, standing or seated	104
Rib shifter	59
Option 2	**Page**
Pendulum swing front/behind	98 or 99
Back scratcher	108
Push forward, pull back	97
Rotating neck massage	91
De-stress your neck	87
Neck settling movements × 3	81

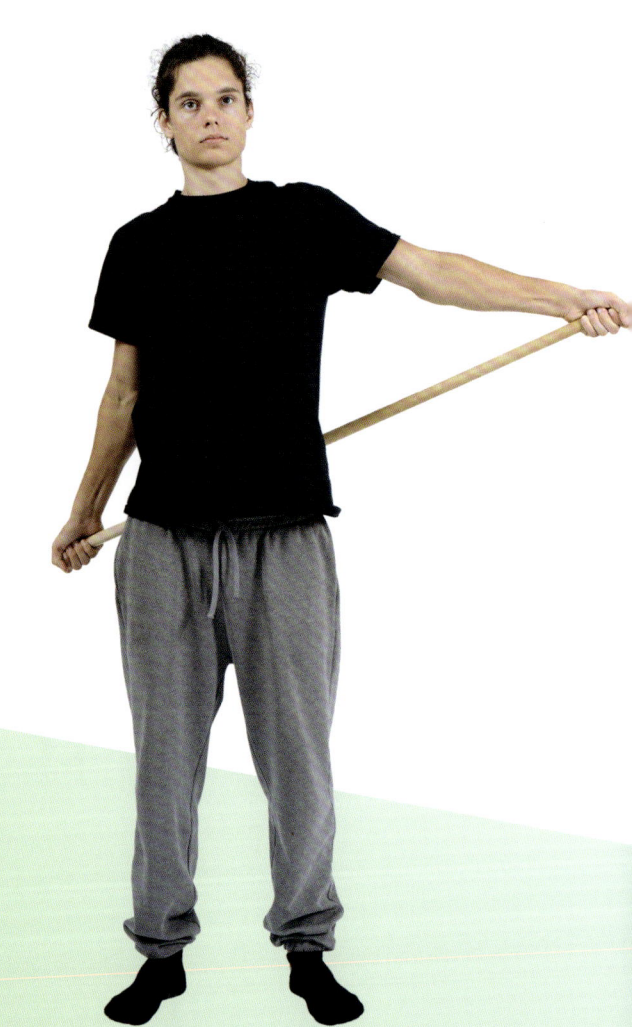

TARGETED EXERCISE COMBINATIONS

For the gardener option 1

Chest lift
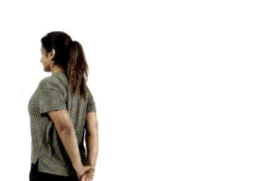

Chest and shoulder release A or B
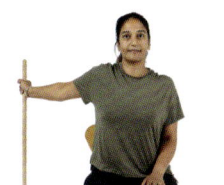

Horizontal arm circles
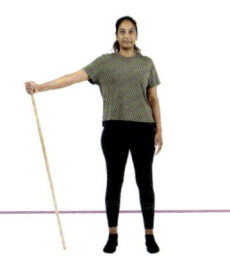

Upper back massage
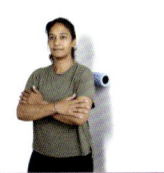

One-arm forward hang, standing or seated
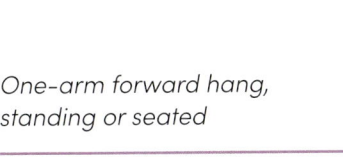

Rib shifter
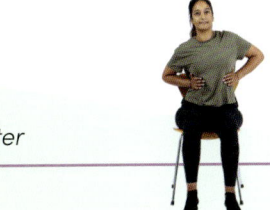

For the gardener option 2

Pendulum swing front/behind
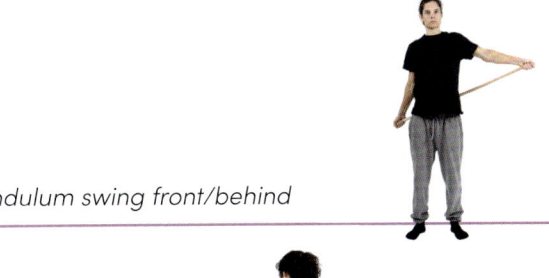

Back scratcher
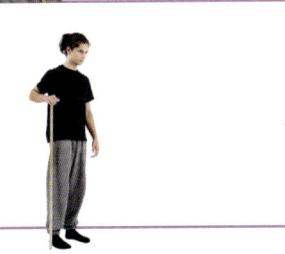

Push forward, pull back
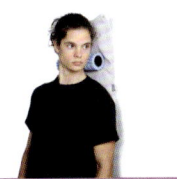

Rotating neck massage
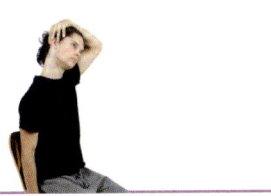

De-stress your neck

Neck settling movements × 3
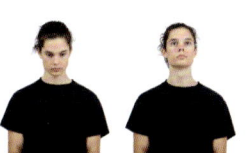

For people who do creative hobbies, such as artists, crafters, crocheters, sewers and knitters

Crafters do many hours of fine motor skills in one position. This results in the upper body becoming stiff and uncomfortable. People who enjoy these hobbies need to take regular movement breaks to maintain comfort and to be free to enjoy their activities without pain. Below you will find a couple of movement medicine options for you to do every hour to keep you happily crafting.

Choose one of the following options (or try both!) after doing the essential warm-up movements in table 9.1 (*see* p. 116):

Table 9.16

Option 1	Page
Cross-body reach	100
Desk chest stretch	69
Rib shifter	59
Nodding neck massage or rotating neck massage	90 or 91
One-arm forward hang, standing or seated	104
Upper back easer A	60
Option 2	**Page**
Put your coat on	101
Back scratcher	108
Horizontal arm circles	96
Upper back massage	75
De-stress your neck	87
Neck settling movements × 3	81

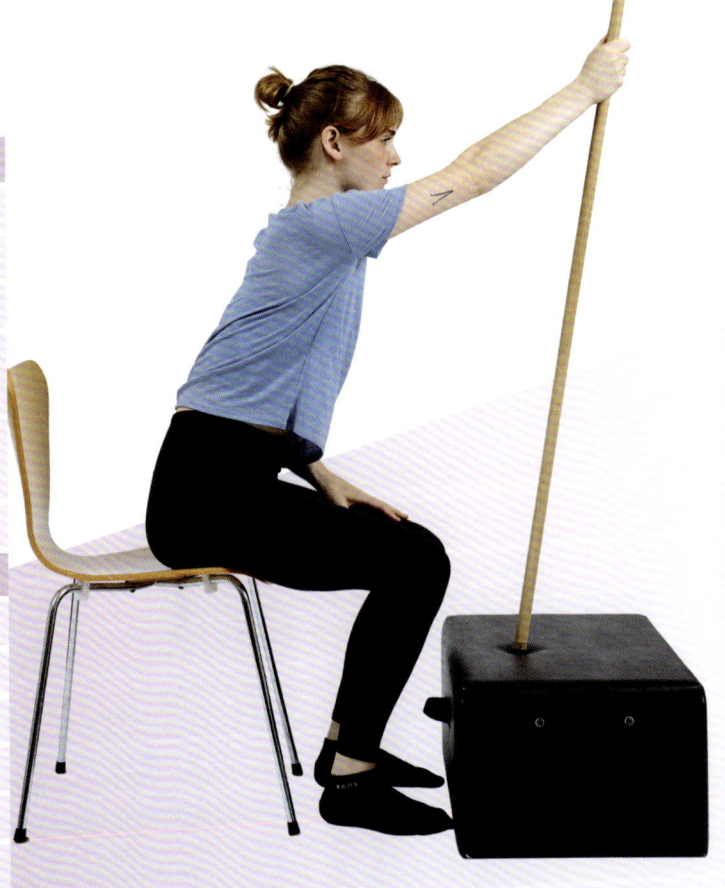

TARGETED EXERCISE COMBINATIONS

For people who do creative hobbies option 1

Cross-body reach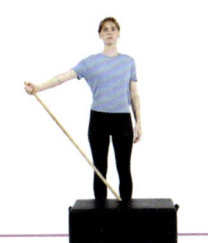

Desk chest stretch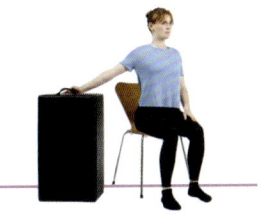

Rib shifter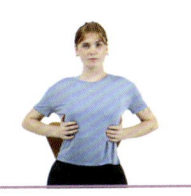

Nodding neck massage or rotating neck massage

One-arm forward hang, standing or seated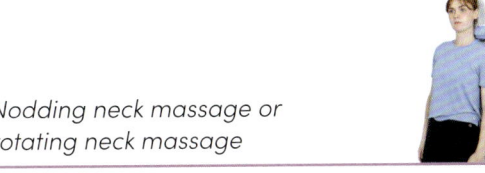

Upper back easer A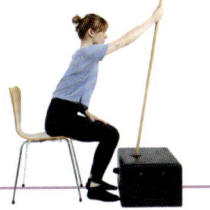

For people who do creative hobbies option 2

Put your coat on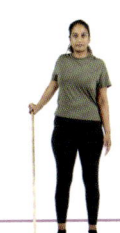

Back scratcher

Horizontal arm circles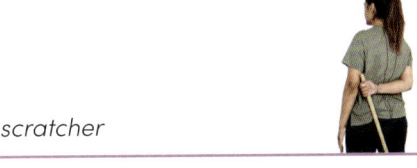

Upper back massage

De-stress your neck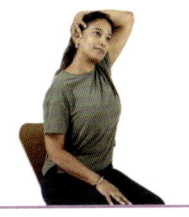

Neck settling movements × 3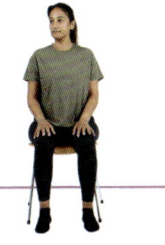

147

MAKE MOVEMENT YOUR MEDICINE

For the cyclist

It can be challenging to maintain good upper body posture when you're cycling, because you need to lean your upper back forwards to reach the handle bars, and lifting your head to look forwards and around compresses the neck. Many cyclists develop a rounded upper back, rounded shoulders and forward head posture, which puts them at risk of developing aches and pains. The answer is to perform exercises regularly to counteract the compressive effects of cycling on the upper body. Our suggestions can be tried in sequence or any one can be done at any time.

Choose one of the following options (or try both!) after doing the essential warm-up movements in table 9.1 (see p. 116):

Table 9.17

Option 1	Page
Two-arm swipe	67
Side hang, standing or seated	106
Push forward, pull back	97
Lying down neck massage	92
Release your neck	89
Neck saucer glide	84 |//
Option 2	Page
Pendulum swing, front or behind	98 or 99
Chest and shoulder release A or B	72 or 73
Upper back easer A	60
Top of shoulder massage	112
Back of neck stretch A	85
Neck settling movements × 3	81

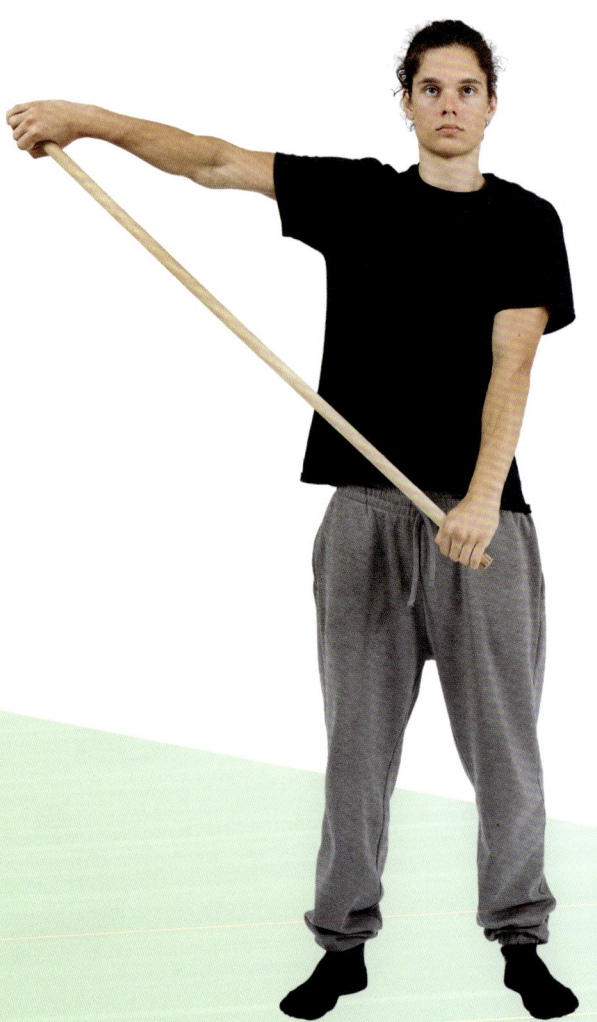

TARGETED EXERCISE COMBINATIONS

For the cyclist option 1

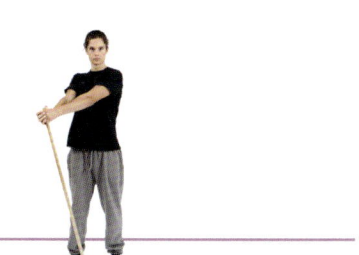
Two-arm swipe

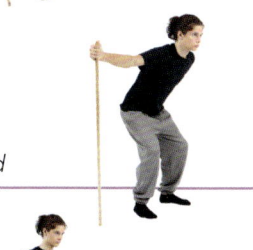
Side hang, standing or seated

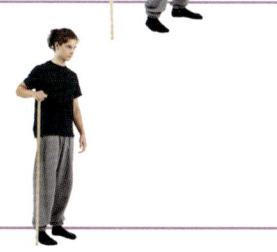
Push forward, pull back

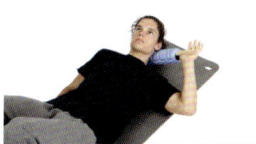
Lying down neck massage

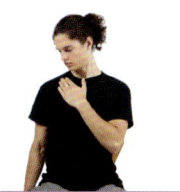
Release your neck

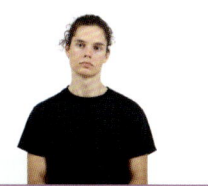
Neck saucer glide

For the cyclist option 2

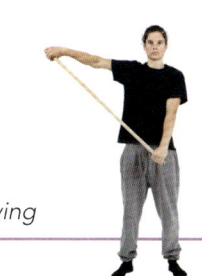
Pendulum swing

Chest and shoulder release A or B

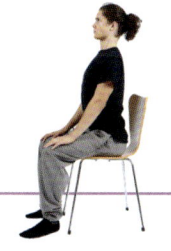
Upper back easer A

Top of shoulder massage

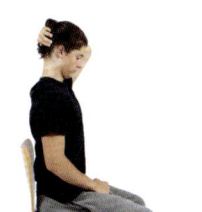
Back of neck stretch A

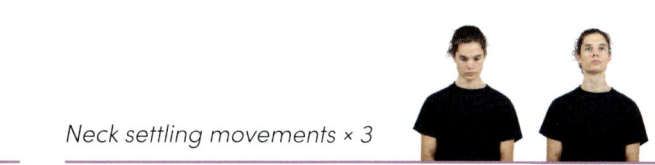
Neck settling movements × 3

For the runner

Most runners tend to be concerned with lower body problems such as knee injuries, but poor function in the upper body can have a big effect on running. If your upper back is stiff, with poor rotation, this can lead to knee and hip problems as well as a painful neck and shoulders.

Choose one of the following options (or try both!) after doing the essential warm-up movements in table 9.1 (*see* p. 116):

Table 9.18

Option 1	Page
Upper back easer B	68
Side hang, standing or seated	106
Horizontal arm circles	96
Shoulder blade muscle massage	111
Two-arm forward hang, seated	71
Rib shifter	59

Option 2	Page
Two-arm swipe	67
Decompress your neck	88
Neck settling movements × 3	81
Lying down neck massage	92
Chest and shoulder release A or B	72 or 73
Upper back easer A	60

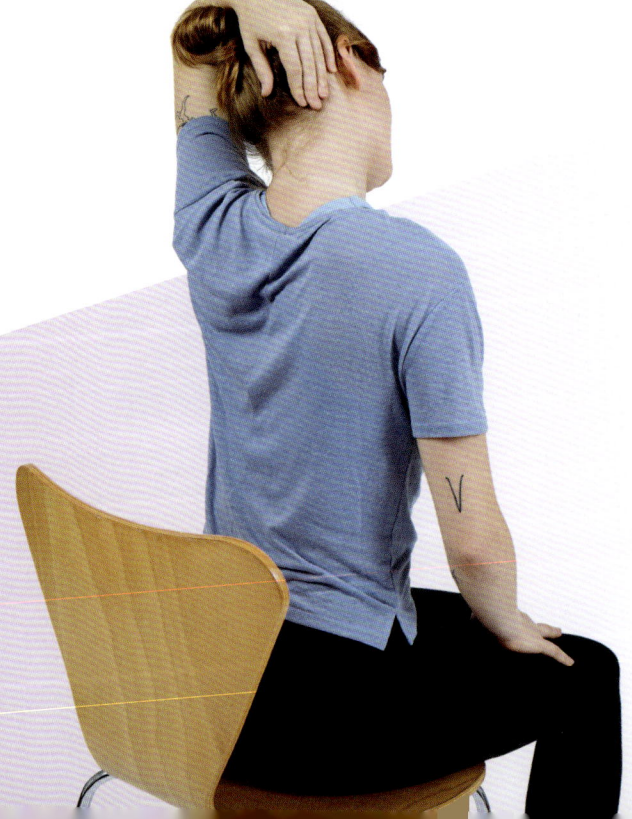

TARGETED EXERCISE COMBINATIONS

For the runner option 1

Upper back easer B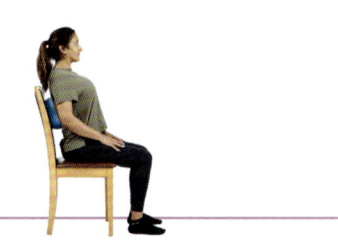

Side hang, standing or seated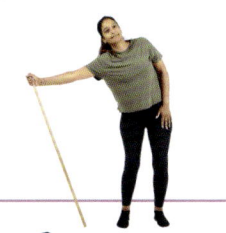

Horizontal arm circles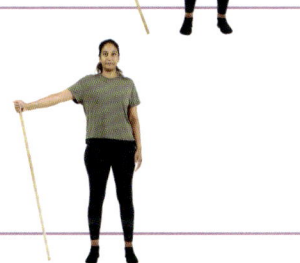

Shoulder blade muscle massage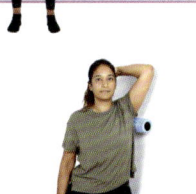

Two-arm forward hang, seated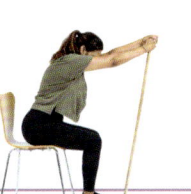

Rib shifter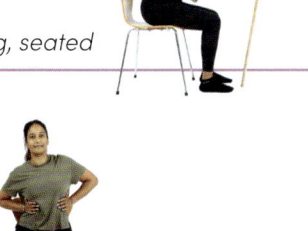

For the runner option 2

Two-arm swipe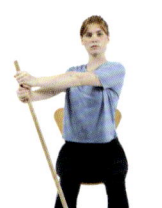

Decompress your neck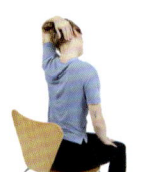

Neck settling movements × 3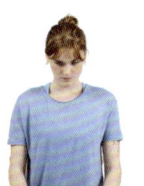

Lying down neck massage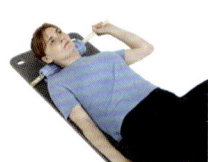

Chest and shoulder release A or B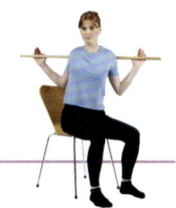

Upper back easer A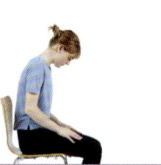

MAKE MOVEMENT YOUR MEDICINE

For the golfer and tennis/padel player

These combinations are useful both before and after playing golf, tennis or indeed any racquet sport. They are also useful as maintenance of the upper body between training sessions or competitions. To reduce the likelihood of a shoulder injury when playing it is important to keep the upper body mobile and stretched.

Choose one of the following options (or try both!) after doing the essential warm-up movements in table 9.1 (*see* p. 116):

Table 9.19

Option 1	Page
Pendulum swing front/behind	98 or 99
Side hang, standing or seated	106
Horizontal arm circles	96
Shoulder blade muscle massage	111
Across-body hang, standing or seated	105
Cross-body reach	100
Option 2	**Page**
Underarm swing	102
Backward hang	107
Push forward, pull back	97
Shoulder rolling massage or Shoulder cross-fibre massage	109 or 110
One-arm forward hang, standing or seated	104
Horizontal arm circles	96

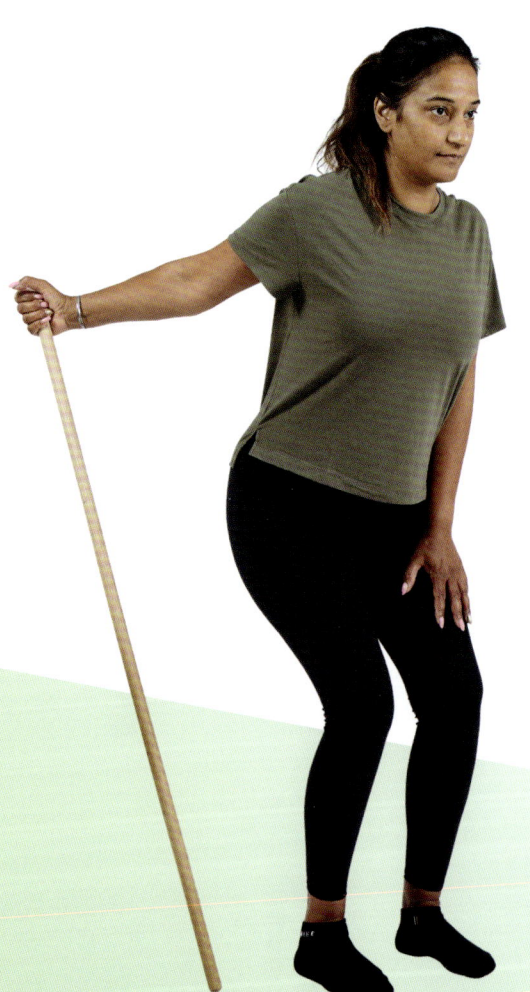

TARGETED EXERCISE COMBINATIONS

For the golfer and tennis/padel player option 1

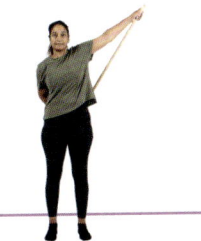

Pendulum swing front/behind

Side hang, standing or seated

Horizontal arm circles

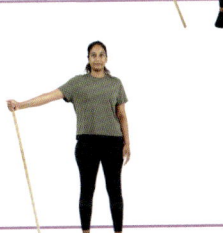

Shoulder blade muscle massage

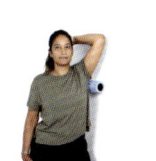
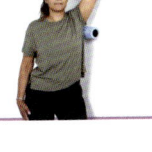

Across-body hang, standing or seated

Cross-body reach

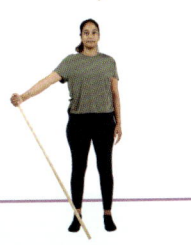

For the golfer and tennis/padel player option 2

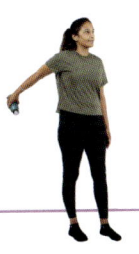

Underarm swing

Backward hang

Push forward, pull back

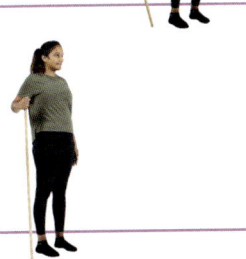

Shoulder rolling massage or Shoulder cross-fibre massage

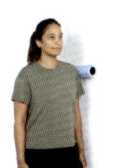

One-arm forward hang, standing or seated

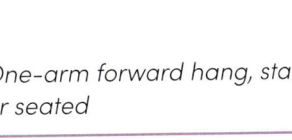
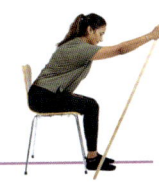

Horizontal arm circles

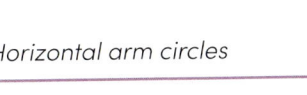

FOR SPECIFIC ISSUES

Do you ache when you first get out of bed? Does your head tend to poke forwards, making your neck ache? Have you ever been shocked by how hunched you look when you see your reflection in a window or mirror? Or have you noticed that you stoop or your shoulders are rounding, very restricted or painful?

These are all common upper body issues and if you recognise any of those symptoms – or simply want to avoid ever experiencing them – we have lots of ideas for ways to combine movements, stretches and self-massages to address them.

Feeling stiff when you first wake up is quite normal and not something to worry about, but it's also great to know what you can do to ease it. The exercise combinations we suggest can be done sitting on your bed or standing near it. The upper back rotation, lying can even be done on your bed, as long as your mattress is firm. Another tip is to leave a pole accessible near your bed, since it will remind you to move.

If the muscles around your upper back, neck and shoulders are really tight, you will find the movements we suggest soothing and helpful, but we always advise you to work in a range of movement that does not cause pain directly in the muscles or joints. Stretches using a pole are particularly good for the upper back and shoulders, but we recommend you follow each of them with a settling movement to soothe and calm the muscles at their new lengths.

Remember to start with the warm-up movements in table 9.1 (*see* p. 116).

Morning stiffness

If you are one of the many people who wake up feeling stiff and achy in their upper back, neck and shoulders, the sequences below can be a welcome help. You will find that they help to loosen tight areas, improve flexibility and relax tight muscles. They make it easier to start your day more comfortably.

Choose one of the following options (or try both!) after doing the essential warm-up movements in table 9.1 (*see* p. 116):

Table 9.20

Option 1	Page
Upper back rotation, lying	63
Back of neck stretch A or B	85 or 86
Neck settling movements × 3	81
Upper back massage	75
One-arm forward hang, standing or seated	104
Rib release	64
Option 2	**Page**
Two-arm swipe	67
Two-arm forward hang, seated	71
Rib shifter	59
Nodding neck massage	90
Rib opener stretch	70
Neck settling movements × 3	81

TARGETED EXERCISE COMBINATIONS

Morning stiffness option 1

Upper back rotation, lying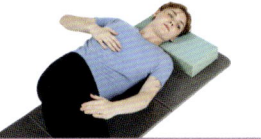

Back of neck stretch A or B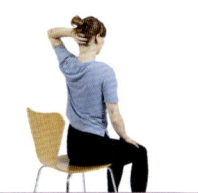

Neck settling movements × 3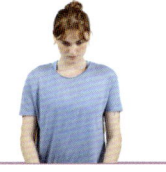

Upper back massage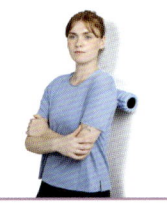

One-arm forward hang, standing or seated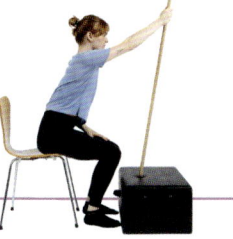

Rib release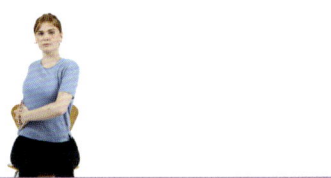

Morning stiffness option 2

Two-arm swipe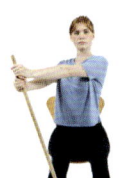

Two-arm forward hang, seated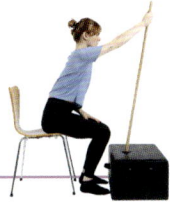

Rib shifter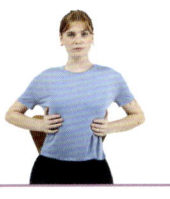

Nodding neck massage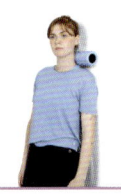

Rib opener stretch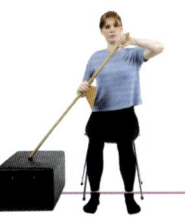

Neck settling movements × 3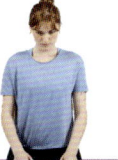

155

Midday reset

These sequences will refresh and revive your upper back, neck and shoulders at lunchtime.

Choose one of the following options (or try both!) after doing the essential warm-up movements in table 9.1 (*see* p. 116):

Table 9.21

Option 1	Page
Upper back rotation, standing, seated or lying	61, 62 or 63
Rib opener stretch	70
Rib shifter	59
Upper back easer A or B	60 or 68
Neck saucer glide	84
Slide the chin in	83
Desk chest stretch	69
Option 2	**Page**
Upper back rotation, standing, seated or lying	61, 62 or 63
Two-arm forward hang, seated	71
Release your neck	89
Neck settling movements × 3	81
Two-arm swipe	67
Upper back round and lift	66
Shoulder blade squeezer	103

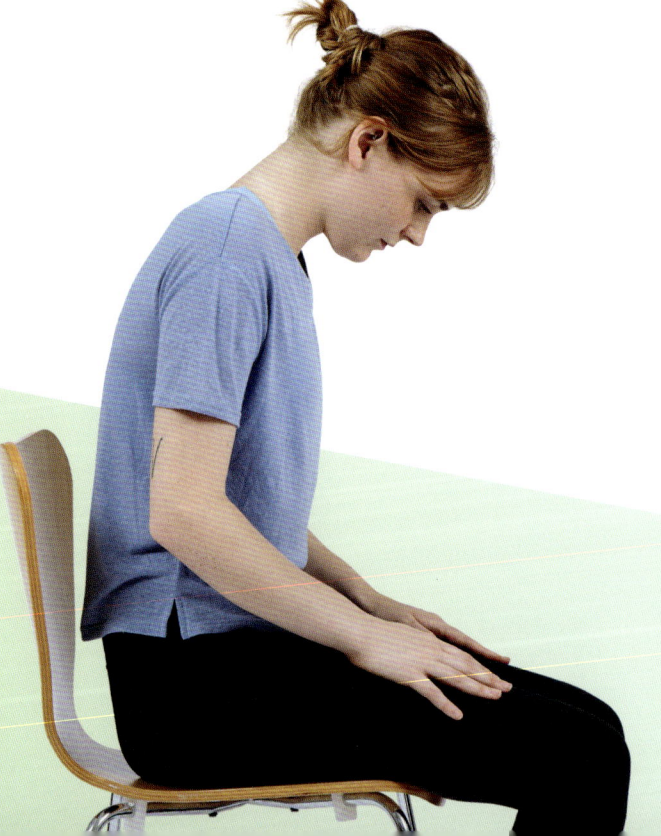

TARGETED EXERCISE COMBINATIONS

Midday reset option 1

Upper back rotation, standing, seated or lying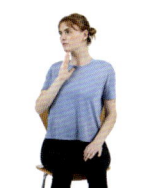

Rib opener stretch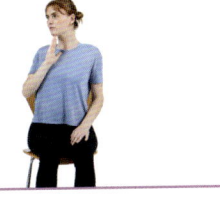

Rib shifter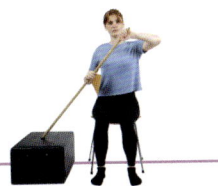

Upper back easer A or B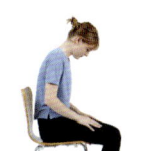

Neck saucer glide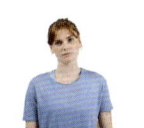

Slide the chin in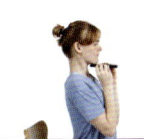

Desk chest stretch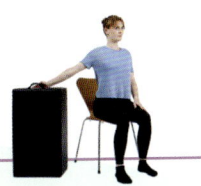

Midday reset option 2

Upper back rotation, standing, seated or lying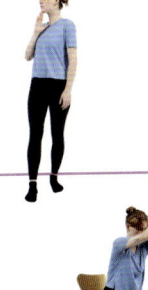

Two-arm forward hang, seated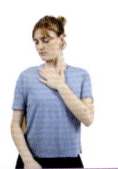

Release your neck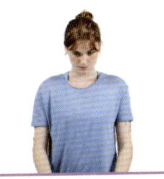

Neck settling movements × 3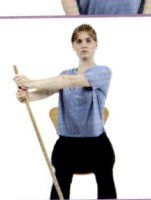

Two-arm swipe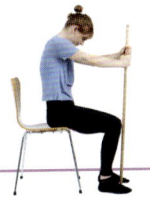

Upper back round and lift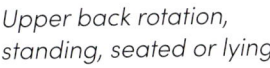

Shoulder blade squeezer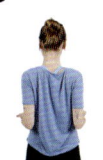

157

Night-time wind-down

To soothe your upper back, neck and shoulders and help you have the best-quality sleep possible, try one or both of the following options. Be sure to adopt a slow, steady pace and maintain regular, relaxed breathing throughout.

As for all the sequences, start by doing the essential warm-up movements in table 9.1 (*see* p. 116):

Table 9.22

Option 1	Page
Upper back rotation, standing, seated or lying	61, 62 or 63
Two-arm forward hang, seated	71
Horizontal arm circles	96
Turn right, turn left	82
Back of the neck stretch A or B	85 or 86
Neck settling movements x 3	81
Rib release	64

Option 2	Page
Chest lift	65
Across-body hang, standing or seated	105
Push forward, pull back	97
Decompress your neck	88
Neck settling movements x 3	81
Two-arm swipe	67
Pendulum swing front or behind	98 or 99

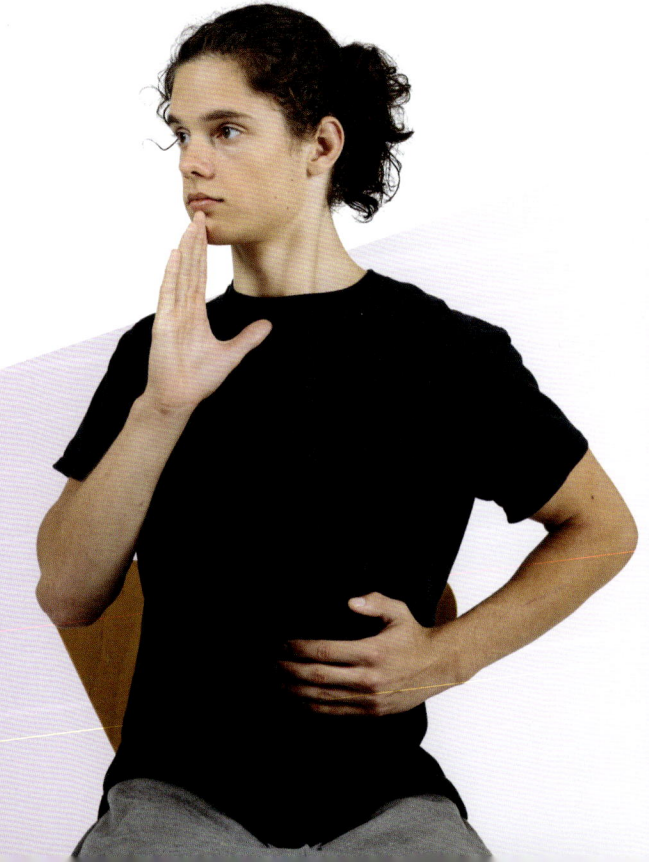

TARGETED EXERCISE COMBINATIONS

Night-time wind-down option 1

Upper back rotation, standing, seated or lying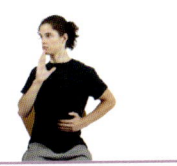

Two-arm forward hang, seated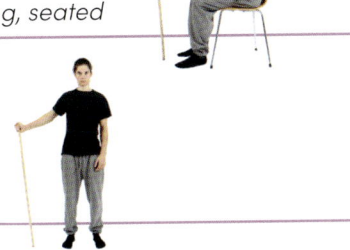

Horizontal arm circles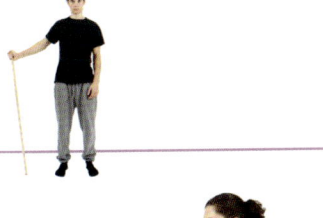

Turn right, turn left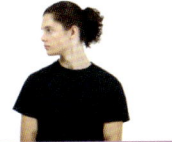

Back of neck stretch A or B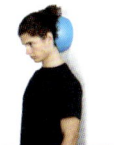

Neck settling movements × 3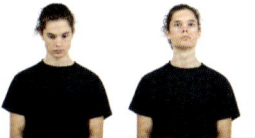

Rib release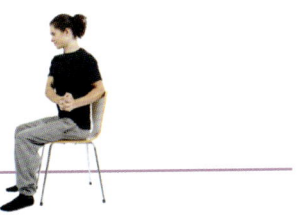

Night-time wind-down option 2

Chest lift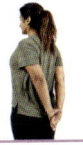

Across-body hang, standing or seated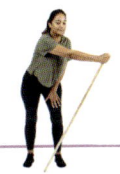

Push forward, pull back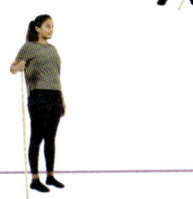

Decompress your neck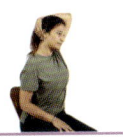

Neck settling movements × 3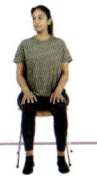

Two-arm swipe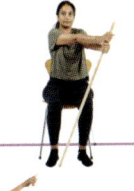

Pendulum swing front or behind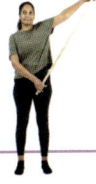

Maintenance sequence

As mentioned, the key upper back movements of flexion/extension, rotation and side bending are the essential foundations for maintaining a well-functioning upper body. The options below include these important exercises, together with a balance of additional ones to give you two sequences for maintaining a healthy upper back, neck and shoulders.

Choose one of the following options (or try both!) after doing the essential warm-up movements in table 9.1 (*see* p. 116):

Table 9.23

Option 1	Page
Upper back easer A	60
Upper back rotation, seated	62
Rib opener stretch	70
Back of neck stretch A or B	85 or 86
Neck saucer glide	84
Two-arm forward hang, standing or seated	71
Rib shifter	59
Option 2	**Page**
Upper back round and lift	66
Upper back rotation, standing	61
Rib opener stretch	70
Release your neck	89
Neck settling movements × 3	81
One-arm forward hang, standing or seated or Side hang, standing or seated	104 or 106
Horizontal arm circles	96

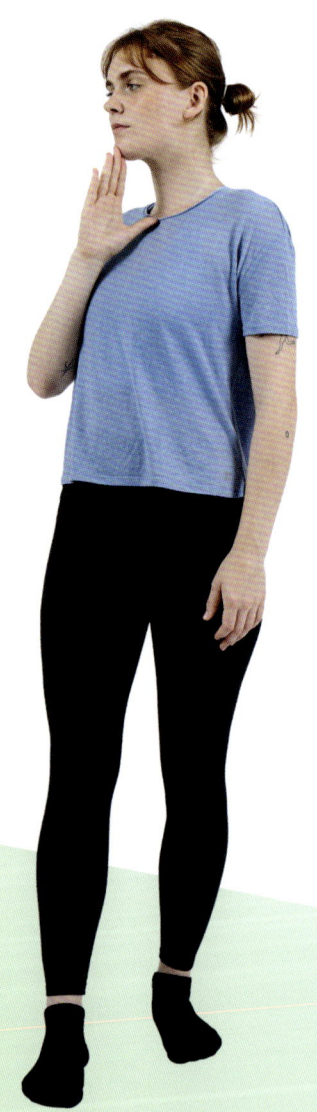

TARGETED EXERCISE COMBINATIONS

Maintenance sequence option 1

Upper back easer A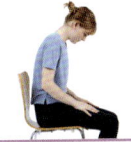

Upper back rotation, seated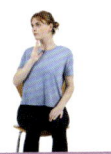

Rib opener stretch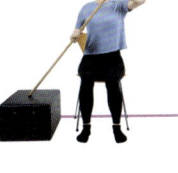

Back of neck stretch A or B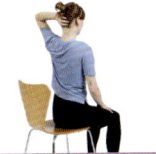

Neck saucer glide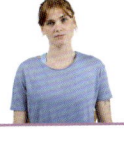

Two-arm forward hang, standing or seated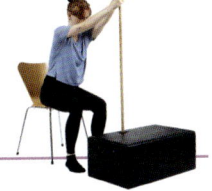

Rib shifter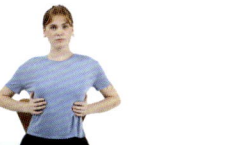

Maintenance sequence option 2

Upper back round and lift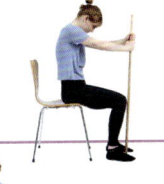

Upper back rotation, standing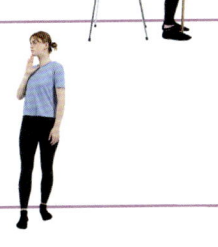

Rib opener stretch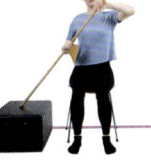

Release your neck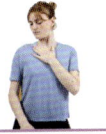

Neck settling movements × 3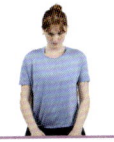

One-arm forward hang, standing or seated or Side hang, standing or seated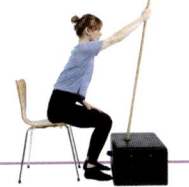

Horizontal arm circles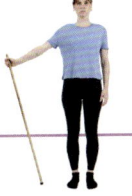

161

MAKE MOVEMENT YOUR MEDICINE

Forward head and neck posture

The sequences below will help you by loosening and opening tight muscles, making it easier to hold your head and neck in a more upright, natural position.

Choose one of the following options (or try both!) after doing the essential warm-up movements in table 9.1 (see p. 116):

Table 9.24

Option 1	Page
Slide the chin in	83
Back of neck stretch A	85
Neck settling movements × 3	81
Nodding neck massage	90
Release your neck	89
Neck saucer glide	84
Option 2	**Page**
Turn right, turn left	82
Desk chest stretch	69
Rib shifter	59
Rotating neck massage	91
De-stress your neck	87
Neck settling movements × 3	81

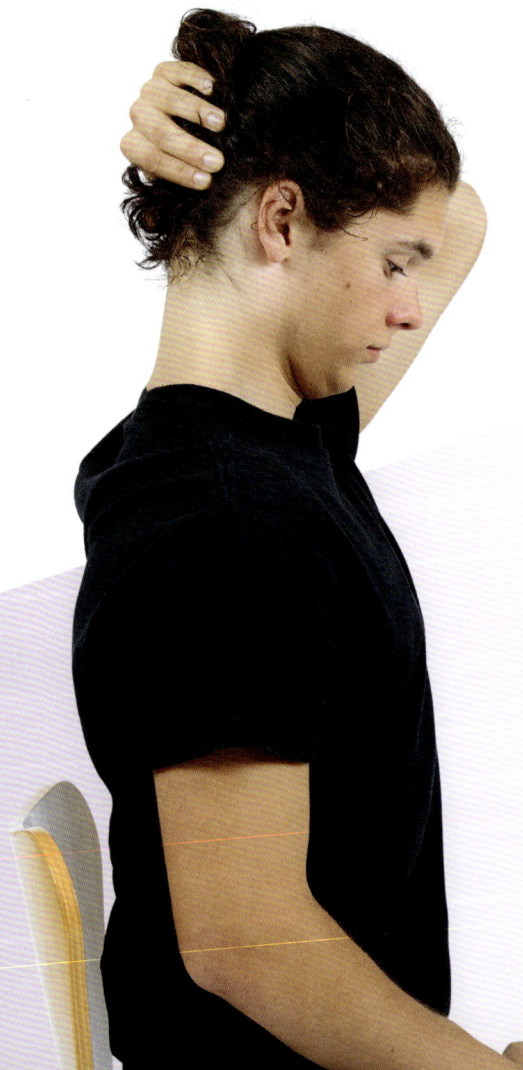

TARGETED EXERCISE COMBINATIONS

Forward head and neck posture option 1

Slide the chin in

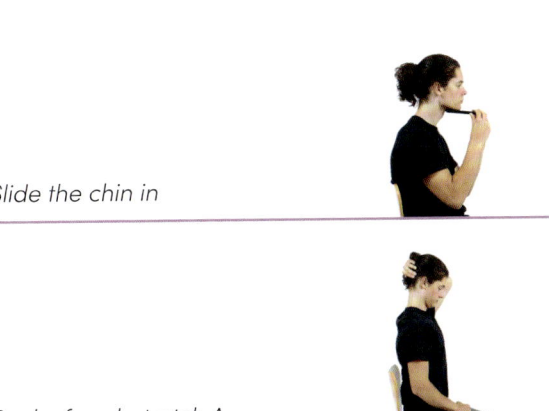

Back of neck stretch A

Neck settling movements × 3

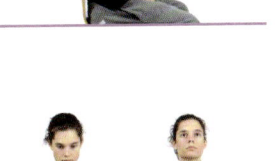

Nodding neck massage

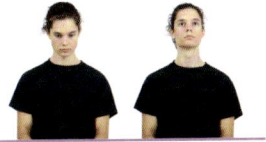

Release your neck

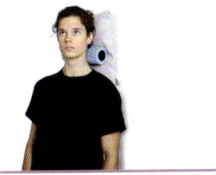

Neck saucer glide

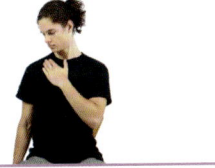

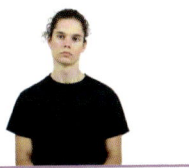

Forward head and neck posture option 2

Turn right, turn left

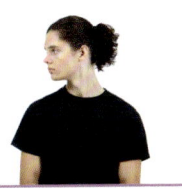

Desk chest stretch

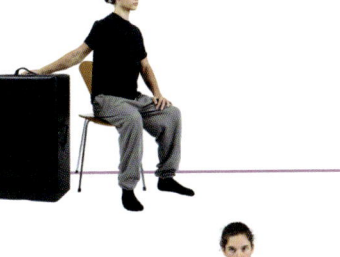

Rib shifter

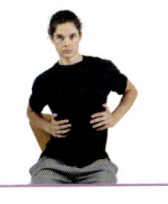

Rotating neck massage

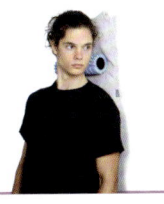

De-stress your neck

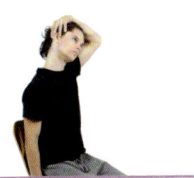

Neck settling movements × 3

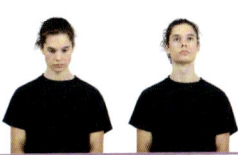

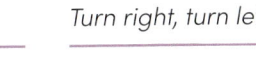

Rounding posture

The movements, stretches and self-massages below will help you by opening and stretching tight muscles and mobilising the spine and upper back. This will help your body to return to a more upright and balanced posture.

Choose one of the following options (or try both!) after doing the essential warm-up movements in table 9.1 (*see* p. 116):

Table 9.25

Option 1	Page
Upper back rotation, lying	63
One-arm forward hang, standing or seated	104
Horizontal arm circles	96
Upper back massage	75
Chest and shoulder release A or B	72 or 73
Rib shifter	59
Option 2	**Page**
Two-arm swipe	67
Desk chest stretch	69
Push forward, pull back	97
Side of back massage	76
Side hang, standing or seated	106
Horizontal arm circles	96

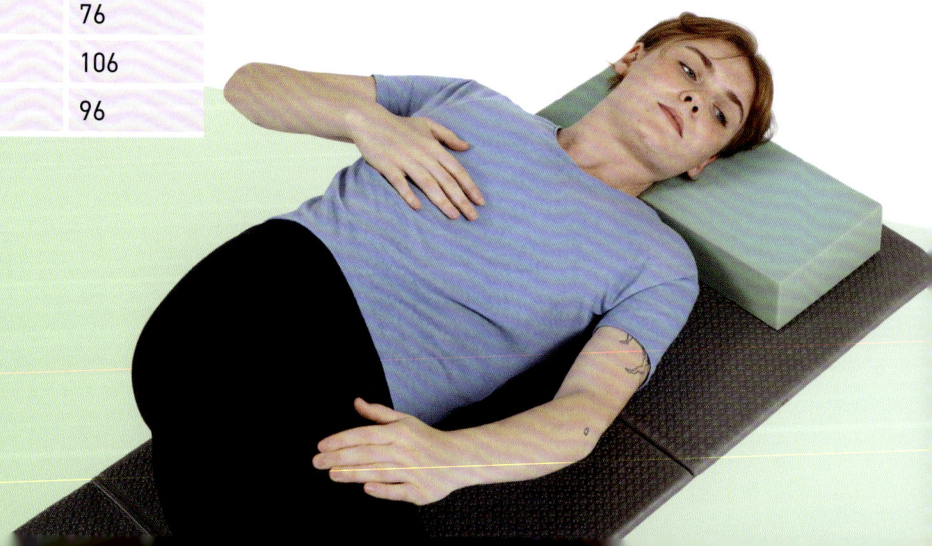

TARGETED EXERCISE COMBINATIONS

Rounding posture option 1

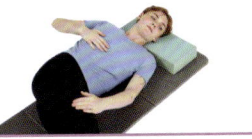
Upper back rotation, lying

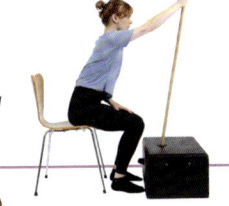
One-arm forward hang, standing or seated

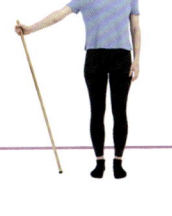
Horizontal arm circles

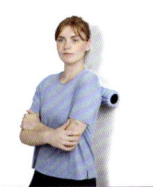
Upper back massage

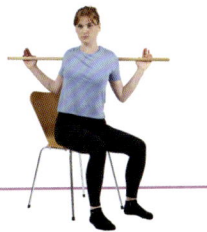
Chest and shoulder release A or B

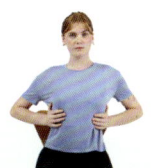
Rib shifter

Rounding posture option 2

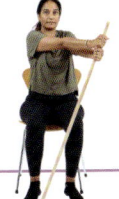
Two-arm swipe

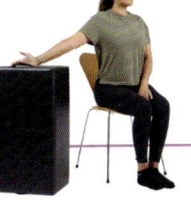
Desk chest stretch

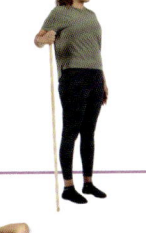
Push forward, pull back

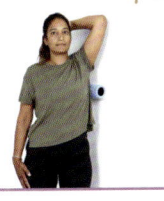
Side of back massage

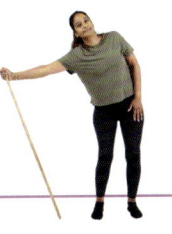
Side hang, standing or seated

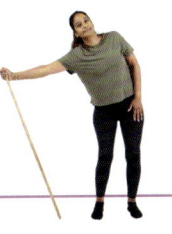
Horizontal arm circles

Arthritic shoulders

These sequences help arthritic shoulders by improving joint mobility, reducing stiffness and improving circulation to the affected tissues. Gentle hanging decompresses the shoulder joint, which can reduce impingement and inflammation. Doing the sequences regularly can decrease pain and improve function.

Choose one of the following options (or try both!) after doing the essential warm-up movements in table 9.1 (see p. 116):

Table 9.26

Option 1	Page
Cross-body reach	100
One-arm forward hang, standing or seated	104
Push forward, pull back	97
Shoulder rolling massage or Cross-fibre massage	109 or 110
Across-body hang standing or seated	105
Underarm swing	102
Option 2	**Page**
Pendulum swing front/behind	98 or 99
Side hang, standing or seated	106
Horizontal arm circles	96
Top of shoulder massage	112
Back scratcher	108
Push forward, pull back	97

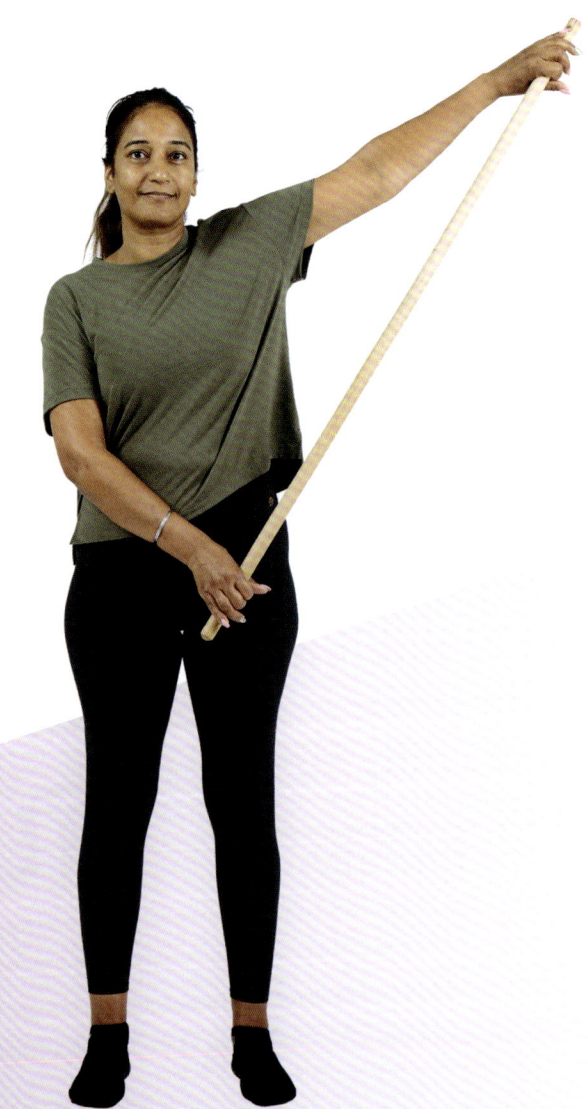

TARGETED EXERCISE COMBINATIONS

Arthritic shoulders option 1

Cross-body reach
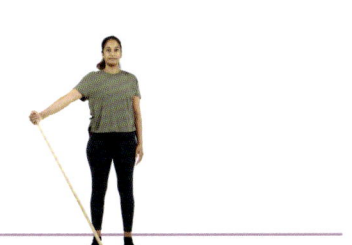

One-arm forward hang, standing or seated
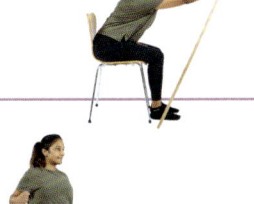

Push forward, pull back
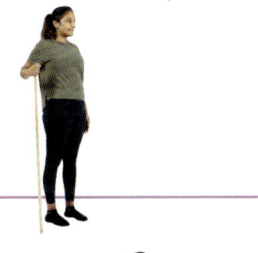

Shoulder rolling massage or Cross-fibre massage
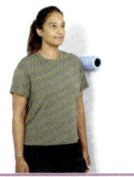

Across-body hang, standing or seated
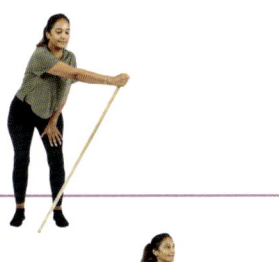

Underarm swing
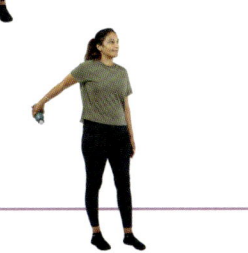

Arthritic shoulders option 2

Pendulum swing front/behind
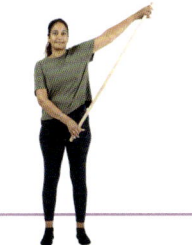

Side hang standing or seated
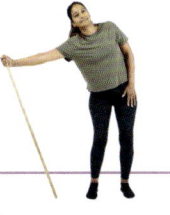

Horizontal arm circles
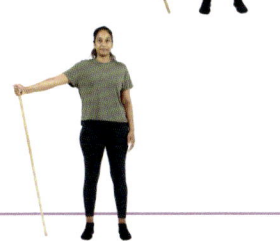

Top of shoulder massage
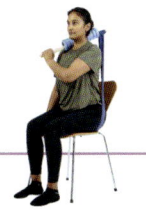

Back scratcher
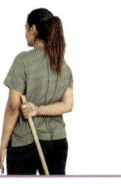

Push forward, pull back
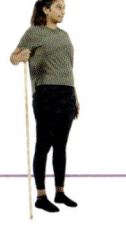

For the natural wear and tear from ageing

As we get older, the likelihood of aches and pains increases because of the natural and gradual changes in the body. Stooping and stiffness are two of the most common signs of this, so to help you to stand tall and move more freely, be sure to include movement as medicine in your daily routine.

Choose one of the following options (or try both!) after doing the essential warm-up movements in table 9.1 (*see* p. 116):

Table 9.27

Option 1	Page
Shoulder blade squeezer	103
One-arm forward hang, standing or seated	104
Horizontal arm circles	96
Upper back massage	75
Side hang, standing or seated	106
Two-arm swipe	67
Option 2	**Page**
Slide the chin in	83
Desk chest stretch	69
Rib release	64
Shoulder rolling massage or Cross-fibre massage	109 or 110
Two-arm forward hang, seated	71
Upper back easer A	60

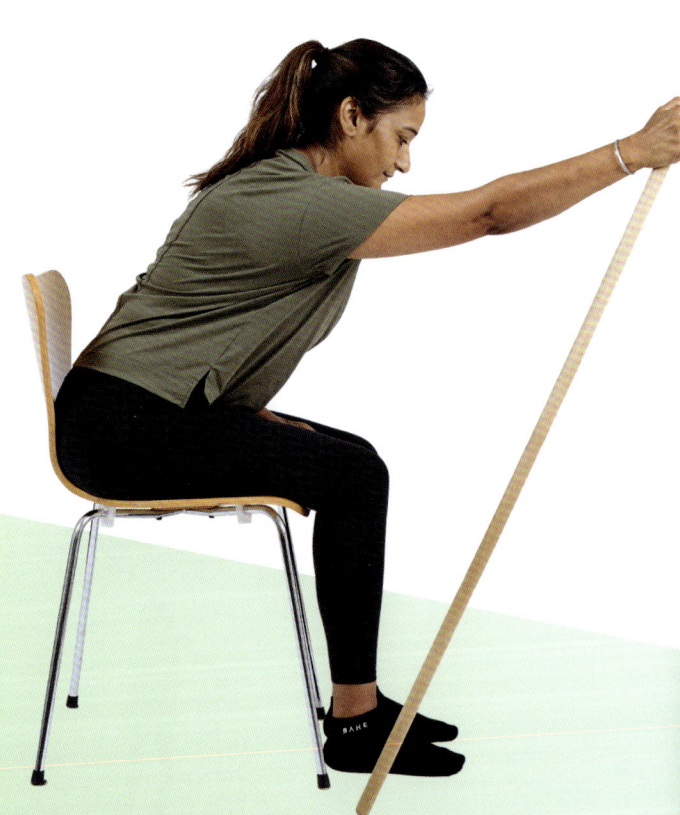

TARGETED EXERCISE COMBINATIONS

For the natural wear and tear from ageing option 1

Shoulder blade squeezer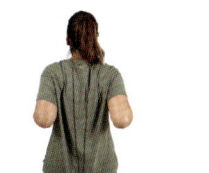

One-arm forward hang, standing or seated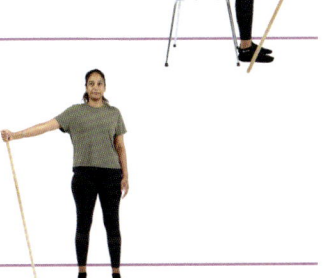

Horizontal arm circles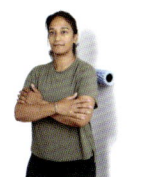

Upper back massage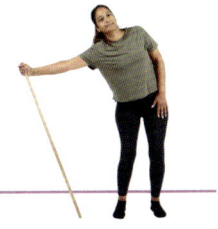

Side hang, standing or seated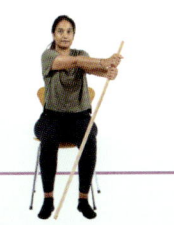

Two-arm swipe

For the natural wear and tear from ageing option 2

Slide the chin in

Desk chest stretch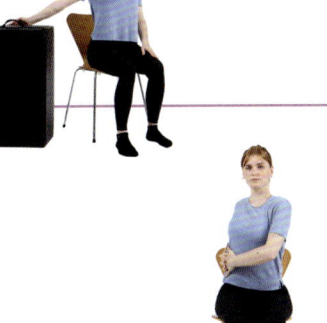

Rib release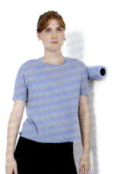

Shoulder rolling massage or Cross-fibre massage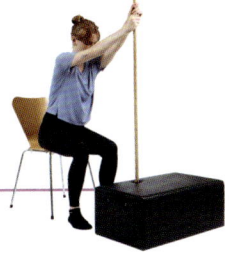

Two-arm forward hang, seated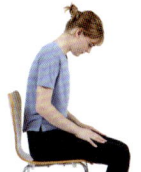

Upper back easer A

169

Dowager's hump; (bump at the base of the neck)

If you spend a lot of time constantly looking down at your phone or using tech, you can develop poor posture from hunching forward. The resulting head forward posture and muscle imbalance from this can cause you to develop a bump at the base of your neck and skin creases in the back of your neck.

To help to prevent or treat this, choose one of the following options (or try both!) after doing the essential warm-up movements in table 9.1 (*see* p. 116):

Table 9.28

Option 1	Page
Chest lift	65
Two-arm forward hang, seated	71
Rib shifter	59
Upper back massage	75
Release your neck	89
Neck settling movements × 3	81
Option 2	**Page**
Neck saucer glide	84
Rib opener stretch	70
Upper back easer B	68
Top of shoulder massage	112
Decompress your neck	88
Neck settling movements × 3	81

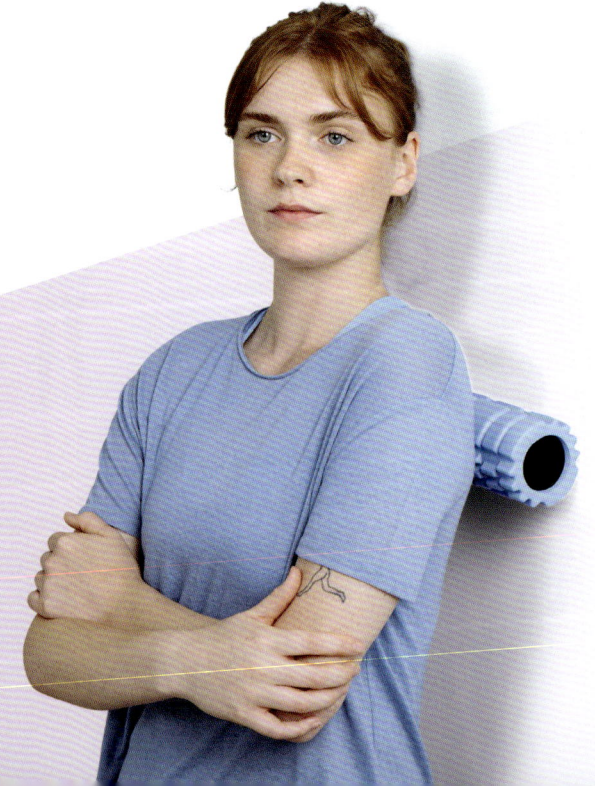

TARGETED EXERCISE COMBINATIONS

Dowager's hump option 1

Chest lift

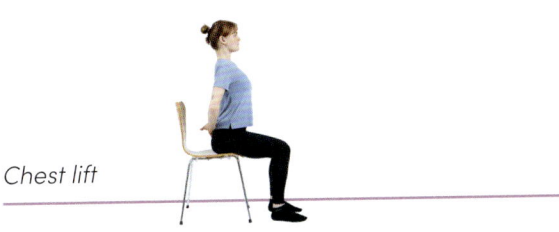

Two-arm forward hang, seated

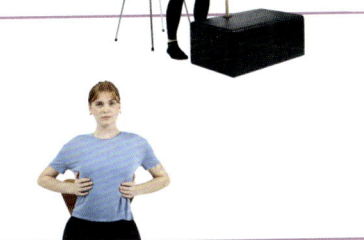

Rib shifter

Upper back massage

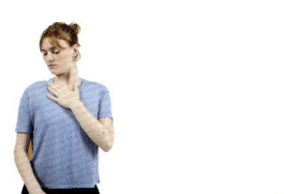

Release your neck

Neck settling movements × 3

Dowager's hump option 2

Neck saucer glide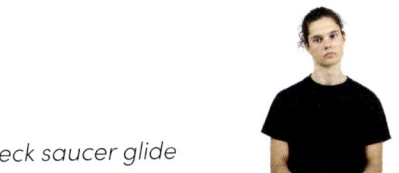

Rib opener stretch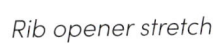

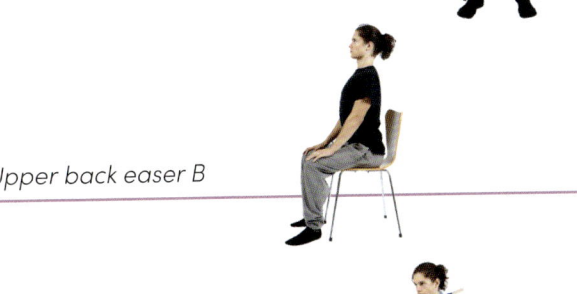

Upper back easer B

Top of shoulder massage

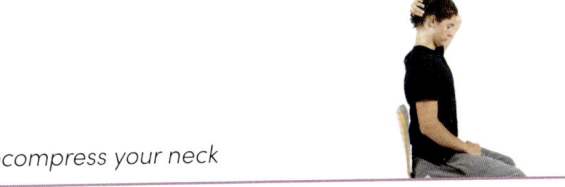

Decompress your neck

Neck settling movements × 3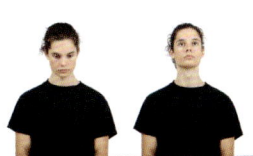

GLOSSARY

Cervical spine: The part of the spine in the neck region, consisting of seven vertebrae.

Cross-fibre massage: A massage technique where pressure is applied across or perpendicular to the muscle fibres.

Diaphragm: The primary muscle used for breathing, located beneath the lungs.

Facet joints: Small joints located between and behind adjacent vertebrae that allow for spinal movement.

Fascia: Connective tissue that surrounds muscles, organs and other structures in the body.

Forward head posture: A condition where the head is positioned in front of the shoulders instead of directly over them.

Ligaments: Tough, fibrous connective tissues that connect bones to other bones, providing stability to joints.

Make Movement Your Medicine: The method described in this book for incorporating movements, stretches and self-massage into daily life.

Neutral posture: The most natural alignment of the body that puts the least amount of strain on muscles and joints.

Pelvic floor muscles: A group of muscles that support the pelvic organs and help control bladder and bowel function.

Roller massage: A self-massage technique using a roller to apply compression and manipulation along muscles.

Rotator cuff: A group of four muscles and their tendons that surround the shoulder joint, providing stability and enabling movement.

Settling movement: A movement that soothes and calms the muscles and joints into their new positions after a stretch.

Tech neck: A modern condition characterised by neck pain and stiffness resulting from prolonged use of electronic devices, particularly with the head bent forwards.

Tendons: Strong, fibrous connective tissues that attach muscles to bones.

Thorax: The part of the body between the neck and the abdomen, containing the ribcage, heart and lungs. For clarity, in this book we use the term upper back to refer to the thorax.

ABOUT US

Andy has an osteopathy degree from The British School of Osteopathy in London, which is complemented by an engineering degree from the University of Sheffield. He is respected as an outstanding osteopath by clients, consultants and other medical practitioners.

Rachel holds a degree in human movement from the University of Wales, and California State University, Long Beach, and a teaching diploma from the University of Reading. This led to her appointment as the body coach to the late Dilys Price OBE, who set the Guinness World Record as the oldest solo woman skydiver. Rachel's emphasis on individual attention for all her clients ensures they achieve their goals – and often more. She also uses her keen sense of fun to guide and coach people.

We have a shared passion for helping people to live free from joint or muscle pain and to learn how to take care of their bodies. To this end, we developed our unique Make Movement Your Medicine method and designed a unique Mobility and Massage pole, a self-help tool called the Adjuvo™ to assist people with exercise therapy at home, work or away. We meet many clients in our private centre in Buckinghamshire, and travel to teach and train other practitioners.

This book represents a continuation of our mission to share our knowledge. We hope you in turn tell others about what you have learned, so they can benefit, too. If during or after dipping into the book you have any queries, please do contact us at breakspearclinic@osteopilates.co.uk

Thank you for reading!

Andy & Rachel Breakspear

THE ADJUVO™ MASSAGE AND MOBILITY POLE

To help us in our work, we developed a unique mobility and self-massage tool for whole-body health and recovery. The Adjuvo™ Mobility and Massage Tool is a versatile all-in-one recovery device designed to improve your range of motion, relieve tension and enhance your muscle and fascial health.

Perfect for fixing hunched posture, pre-workout activation and post-workout recovery, and to relieve general aches and pains.

Lightweight but strong, it is built from high-grade carbon fibre. The Adjuvo™ being bi-telescopic extends from the length of a tennis racket to over 1.8m (6ft) and adjusts to any length in between for precision use and individual requirement.

The Adjuvo™ gives you fast professional relief at home, at work or when training.

If you would like to purchase an Adjuvo™ pole, please visit our website: osteopilates.co.uk

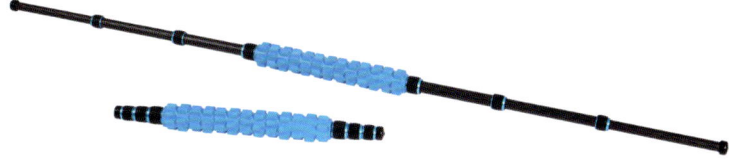

DIRECTORY OF MOVEMENTS, STRETCHES AND SELF-MASSAGES

Across-body hang, standing or seated	p. 105
Back of neck stretch A	p. 85
Back of neck stretch B	p. 86
Back scratcher	p. 108
Backward hang	p. 107
Chest and shoulder release A	p. 72
Chest and shoulder release B	p. 73
Chest lift	p. 65
Cross-body reach	p. 100
De-stress your neck	p. 87
Decompress your neck	p. 88
Desk chest stretch	p. 69
Horizontal arm circles	p. 96
Lying down neck massage	p. 92
Neck saucer glide	p. 84
Neck settling movements x 3	p. 81
Nodding neck massage	p. 90
One-arm forward hang, standing or seated	p. 104
Pendulum swing behind	p. 99
Pendulum swing front	p. 98
Push forward, pull back	p. 97
Put your coat on	p. 101
Release your neck	p. 89
Rib opener stretch	p. 70
Rib release	p. 64
Rib shifter	p. 59
Rotating neck massage	p. 91
Shoulder blade muscle massage	p. 111
Shoulder blade squeezer	p. 103
Shoulder cross-fibre massage	p. 110
Shoulder rolling massage	p. 109
Side hang, standing or seated	p. 106
Side of back massage	p. 76
Slide the chin in	p. 83
Spinal muscle massage	p. 74
Top of shoulder massage	p. 112
Turn right, turn left	p. 82
Two-arm forward hang, seated	p. 71
Two-arm swipe	p. 67
Underarm swing	p. 102
Upper back easer A	p. 60
Upper back easer B	p. 68
Upper back massage	p. 75
Upper back rotation, lying	p. 63
Upper back rotation, seated	p. 62
Upper back rotation, standing	p. 61
Upper back round and lift	p. 66

DIRECTORY OF EXERCISE COMBINATIONS

Essential warm-up exercises — p. 116

Quick sequences
Upper back — p. 118
Neck — p. 120
Shoulders — p. 122

Longer sequences
Upper back — p. 124
Neck — p. 126
Shoulders — p. 128

Combinations for different scenarios:
For the office worker — p. 130
For someone standing on their feet all day — p. 132
For tradespeople and DIYers — p. 134
For musicians and singers — p. 136
For the new parent or grandparent — p. 138
For the traveller — p. 140
For the gamer — p. 142
For the gardener — p. 144
For creative hobbies such as artists, crafters, crocheters, sewers and knitters — p. 146
For the cyclist — p. 148
For the runner — p. 150
For the golfer/tennis/padel player — p. 152

Combinations for specific issues:
Morning stiffness — p. 154
Midday reset — p. 156
Night-time wind down — p. 158
Maintenance sequence — p. 160
Forward head and neck posture — p. 162
Rounding posture — p. 164
Arthritic shoulders — p. 166
Natural wear and tear from ageing — p. 168
Dowagers Hump (bump at the base of the neck) — p. 170

ACKNOWLEDGEMENTS

With love to our children

To our patients and exercise group members; your commitment to our Breakspear Make Movement Your Medicine method is the heartbeat of this book.

Thank you to Commissioning Editor Holly Jarrald and to Sarah Skipper for believing in this book from the beginning and for exceptional guidance. To Lisa Hughes for her initial help and the cover design team at Bloomsbury. Thanks also to Sian and Emil at D.R ink for the beautiful page design.

Thanks to photographer Henry Hunt, models Jay Hoonjan, Tyler Hazell and Lily Little.
And to BAHE Flow for the female models luxury clothing.

Gratitude to the following for their knowledge and support:
Rugby legend George Gregan
Dr Mia Murray
Consultant surgeon Francisco Garcia Rocha
Dr Kim Winser OBE

Special mention to Joan and John Wade for their wisdom, support and Joan's exceptional help completing this book.

Southern California friends Jill and Micheal Pless, thanks for backing and supporting our Adjuvo tool creation.

Little Mimi, our darling dog companion.
All dear friends and close family, thank you for reminding us of the importance of sharing our knowledge across the world, enabling people as they age, to stay feeling younger.

Finally to you, our readers, thank you for picking up this book and for sharing it.

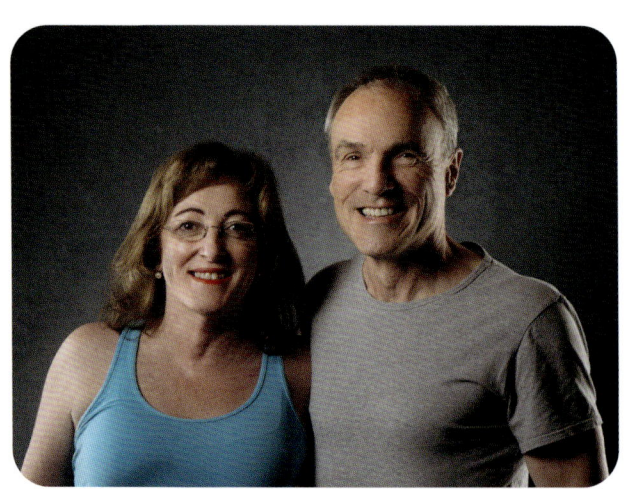